HER
DOWN
THERE

A Guide to Keeping Her Healthy, Happy, and Hydrated.

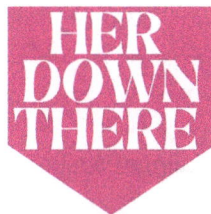

HER DOWN THERE

Letrice Mason MSN, APRN, FNP-C

Letrice Mason MSN, APRN, FNP-C, Author

Www.herdownthere.com

Her Down There: A Guide to Keeping Her Healthy, Happy, and Hydrated.

ISBN: 979-8-218-81028-3 (Paperback)

ISBN: 979-8-218-81721-3 (Hardcover)

Publishing Logistics, Auketria Manor

Www.Themanordigital.com

Cover Design by Jessica Kalinga-Walker

www.Mybrandingstrategist.com

Contents

Introduction

*L*adies let's have a real talk about our hoo-has! For too long, conversations about vaginal health have been all hushed voices and awkward euphemisms. Well, consider this your formal invitation to break out of that stuffy silence and get loud and proud about pH levels, discharge colors, and all things vag.

In this book, we're creating a judgment-free girl gang devoted to celebrating the highs, lows, and hilarious in-betweens of owning a vagina-out with the shame and taboos - with wit, wisdom, and wild sentido humor!

So, all aboard the Vagina Monologues party bus, friends! From the mysteries of menstrual cycles to the wonders of bacterial balance, we're taking a wild ride through every nook and cranny of the female anatomy. And yes, we mean that literally.

This isn't some boring old textbook either, ladies. We're talking juicy storytelling, fascinating science, and enough laugh-out-loud moments to make even your tampon blush. So whether you're a total vagina veteran or just getting your feet wet (pun intended!), there's something in here for everybody.

Ready to dive in and celebrate the power of p*ssy? Then let's do this! It's time to shatter the silence and embrace vaginal vitality in all its funny, fierce, and funky glory. We got this, queens. Now, where's the wine?

What's That Smell? Understanding Vaginal Odors And pH Levels

A healthy vagina is like a flourishing garden - it prospers when nurtured with proper care and attention.

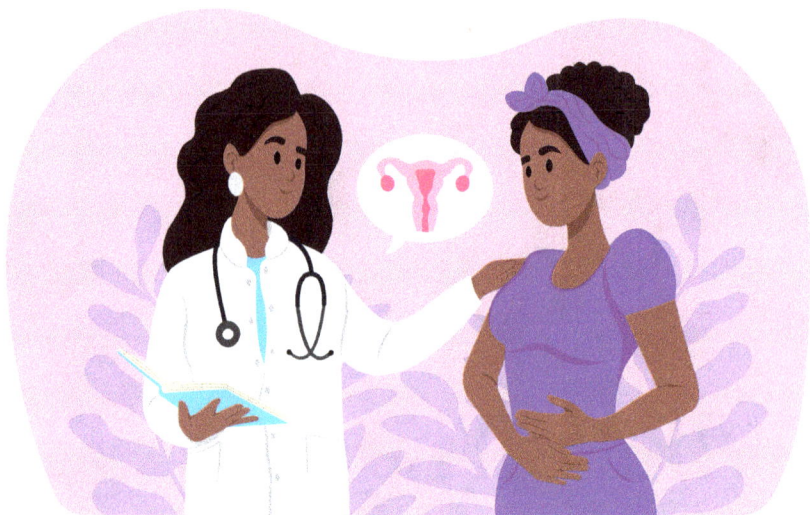

Sarah Jennings lived a life peppered with the kind of misadventures you'd expect in a sitcom. At 29, she had mastered the art of finding humor in the mundane, turning every mishap into a laughable moment for her burgeoning social media following. Sarah's life was a series of comically unfortunate events from accidentally dyeing her cat pink to sending an embarrassingly mushy text meant for her crush to her boss.

On a particularly sunny Tuesday, Sarah encountered what she initially thought was the universe's latest prank on her: a mysterious and decidedly unpleasant odor that seemed to follow her wherever she went. After sniffing around like a detective with a cold, she traced the source to, of all places, her own body. The realization hit her with the subtlety of a sitcom laugh track. "Great," she muttered, "I've officially become a walking, talking punchline."

Determined to solve the mystery with her usual optimism and self-deprecation, Sarah embarked on what she called "Operation Odor Obliteration." Her first step was to conduct an online search, which led to more confusion thanks to the bewildering array of advice ranging from the plausible to the downright bizarre. "According to Dr. Internet, I either have a rare tropical disease or I'm a cheese," Sarah told her followers, trying to mask her growing concern with humor.

The following day, armed with an arsenal of internet-sourced remedies, Sarah transformed her bathroom into a makeshift laboratory. Her first experiment involved a bath concocted from apple cider vinegar, which, according to a blog titled "Smell Fresh, Feel Fresh," promised to balance her pH levels. Clad in a bikini and goggles—for science, of course—Sarah documented the process, trying to stay upbeat. "If this doesn't work, at least I'll make a great salad dressing," she joked, despite the growing worry that her condition might be more serious than she hoped.

Experiment number two was even more outlandish: a homemade garlic paste reputed for its antibacterial properties. The logic was there, but so was the stench. "On the bright side, I'm 100% vampire-proof," Sarah tried to laugh off, even as her eyes watered—not from the garlic fumes, but from the frustration of her failed attempts to find a solution.

Sarah's optimism began to wane with each failed experiment, but her resolve to keep the mood light never faltered. She concocted teas, applied yogurt, and even considered a spell she found on a witchcraft forum, all in the name of science—or, more accurately, desperation.

After her home remedy experiments had proven fruitless—and, in the case of the garlic paste, had added a new layer of complexity to her situation—Sarah decided it was time to seek professional help. The appointment was booked under the disguise of a general check-up, but Sarah knew the true agenda was to solve the mystery of the malodorous malaise that had hijacked her life.

The waiting room was its comedy sketch. Sarah, attempting to appear calm, sat sandwiched between a man who seemed to be practicing bird calls and a woman knitting what appeared to be a sweater for a snake. "I guess we all have our quirks," Sarah mused, trying to ignore the fact that she was about to discuss her vaginal odor with a near stranger.

Dr. Patel, a kind-faced woman with a gentle demeanor, greeted Sarah with a warmth that slightly eased her embarrassment. However, the moment of truth was unavoidably awkward. Sarah stumbled through her explanation, using every euphemism in the book before finally landing on, "My vagina smells funny." Unfazed and ever professional Dr. Patel nodded understandingly, reassuring Sarah that this was a common issue and nothing to be ashamed of.

The diagnosis was bacterial vaginosis, a common condition that many women face but few talk about openly. Dr. Patel explained that it's often related to the balance of bacteria and pH levels in the vagina, and it's nothing that can't be treated with the right medication and care. She emphasized the importance of understanding one's body and not resorting to the "Dr. Internet" approach of self-diagnosis and treatment.

—————————— ♂ ——————————

Sarah's relief was palpable, and she couldn't help but find humor in the situation. "So, you're telling me I don't have a rare cheese disease?" she quipped, finally able to laugh freely about her predicament. Dr. Patel smiled, playing along, "No cheese, just a simple imbalance. And definitely stay away from the garlic."

The mysterious scent that occasionally wafts up from down below – a topic many shy away from but one we're diving into headfirst. Because let's face it, ladies, sometimes our nether regions come with their unique fragrance, and it's not always a bed of roses. But fear not, for we're about to embark on a journey through the fascinating world of vaginal odors and pH levels. Buckle up because things are about to get delightfully scientific!

Exploring pH Levels

So, first things first, what the heck is pH anyway? No, it's not some fancy abbreviation for a spa treatment, although wouldn't that be nice? pH stands for "potential of hydrogen" (not to be confused with a potential hydrogen bomb situation, a different explosion). In simpler terms, pH measures how acidic or basic a solution is.

The vagina is indeed a marvel, often seeming to possess a mind of its own. However, fluctuations in its condition can understandably cause concern of paramount importance to vaginal health i.e. its pH balance. As you may recall from chemistry class, pH signifies the acidity or alkalinity of a substance. Surprisingly, your vaginal pH balance significantly impacts its overall health. An imbalance in pH can manifest in itching or unpleasant odors, potentially indicating issues like yeast infections or bacterial vaginosis.

Vaginal pH serves as a barometer of the acidity or alkalinity of its fluid. When a woman's pH is skewed, she becomes more susceptible to yeast infections, bacterial vaginosis, and potentially sexually transmitted infections, particularly if the vaginal mucosal layer is compromised. The optimal pH typically falls between 3.8 and 4.2, though this range may fluctuate with age and menstrual cycle phase.

For perspective, a pH of 7 denotes neutrality. Below 7 indicates acidity, while above 7 signifies alkalinity. So, picture your vagina akin to acidic tomato juice, diligently maintaining balance and zest. Should you ever sense any imbalance, fear not—provide your pH with the care it warrants, and your vagina will express its gratitude.

What Is A Healthy Vaginal pH Level?

In the realm of women's health, maintaining optimal vaginal pH is paramount. The vagina naturally sustains a slightly acidic environment, typically between 3.8 to 4.5 on the pH scale, serving as a formidable defense against harmful bacteria. However, variations in pH levels occur throughout a woman's life journey.

Throughout the reproductive years, spanning from approximately 14 to 49 years old, women commonly maintain vaginal pH within the healthy range. It's important to note that pH levels may experience a minor uptick before menstruation. Additionally, sexual activity can momentarily raise pH levels to facilitate sperm survival, as sperm thrives in an alkaline environment, reaching 7.0 or even 8.5.

—————————— ♂ ——————————

While a balanced acidic pH during the reproductive years generally translates to reduced infection risk, it may pose conception challenges due to sperm viability. Conversely, post menopause, some women may encounter an elevation in vaginal pH, potentially reaching 7.0. This shift renders post-menopausal women susceptible to infections like bacterial vaginosis (BV) and trichomoniasis, thereby heightening vulnerability to more severe sexually transmitted infections such as HIV or herpes.

How To Know If Your Vaginal Ph Is Off

When the feminine pH balance is disrupted, the female body typically manifests several telltale signs. If any of the following symptoms resonate with you, conducting a home test to gauge your pH levels may be prudent. Should your results fall below 3.8 or exceed 4.5, it's advisable to seek medical attention promptly.

- **Vulvar Discomfort:**

  Persistent itching and swelling of the vulva, beyond what might be attributed to routine factors like shaving or waxing, often indicate a potential infection within the vaginal region.

- **Abnormal Vaginal Discharge:**

  While vaginal discharge can vary in color and consistency, deviations such as a thick, lumpy texture resembling cottage cheese, or hues of yellow, green, or gray, suggest the presence of infection and necessitate a medical consultation.

- **Unpleasant Odor:**

  While every woman's vaginal scent is unique, an unusually strong and offensive odor reminiscent of fish or decaying flesh warrants medical evaluation, especially if accompanied by other symptoms like abnormal discharge.

- **Painful Urination:**

  A burning sensation during urination commonly signifies urinary tract issues, such as infections or kidney stones, necessitating medical evaluation for appropriate management.

- **Discomfort During Intercourse:**

  Experiencing discomfort or burning sensations during intercourse may stem from various factors, including vaginal dryness or underlying infections, warranting medical attention for accurate diagnosis and treatment.

Should you feel uncertain about conducting home tests or interpreting symptoms, seeking guidance from a healthcare professional is advisable. They may conduct further tests, such as pelvic exams or fluid sampling, to ascertain the underlying cause of your symptoms.

Tips For Restoring Your Feminine pH Balance

Restoring your vaginal pH balance naturally involves adopting simple steps and adjusting your lifestyle. Here are some proven methods:

- **Steer Clear of Douching:**

  Instead of resorting to douching or using scented soaps, which can disrupt your pH levels, opt for a gentler approach. Cleanse your intimate area with lukewarm water and unscented soap. Remember, your vagina is adept at self-cleansing, so there's no need to wash inside.

- **Embrace Condom Usage:**

  Condoms serve a dual purpose: safeguarding against sexually transmitted infections and helping maintain optimal vaginal pH levels by countering the alkaline properties of semen. However, be cautious with flavored, pre-lubricated, and spermicidal condoms as they may lead to vaginal irritation and upset the delicate balance.

- **Choose Breathable Clothing:**

  Opt for looser underwear and clothing, especially those made from breathable materials like cotton. Tight synthetic fabrics can create an oppressive environment, promoting bacterial growth. Avoid tight jeans or leggings without a cotton lining to encourage air circulation and reduce the risk of infections.

———————————— ♂ ————————————

Remember to change out of damp attire promptly, whether it's a swimsuit or workout gear, to prevent excess moisture buildup in the vaginal area. By incorporating these practices into your routine, you can effectively rebalance your feminine pH and promote vaginal health naturally.

And there you have it, ladies - So, next time you hear someone talking about pH, you can proudly say, "Oh, you mean the secret sauce that keeps my lady garden flourishing!"

Remember, pH may be a small two-letter word, but it plays a big role in keeping your lady bits happy and healthy. It's like the conductor of your body's orchestra, ensuring that everything stays in perfect harmony. So, treat your vagina like the queen she is, and she'll reward you with smooth sailing down there.

But fear not, for our journey is far from over! In the next chapter, we'll tackle the ever elusive topic of vaginal odors - from the downright funky to the surprisingly sweet. So, grab your nose plugs (just kidding) and join me as we sniff out the truth behind those mysterious smells. Trust me, it's going to be a wild ride!

Until then, keep it pH-fabulous, ladies, and remember: when life gives you lemons, thank your lucky stars. They're not messing with your vaginal pH. Cheers to happy, healthy lady bits, and I'll see you in the next chapter!

Daily Maintenance: Keeping 'Her' Happy

Vaginal health is all about maintaining harmony-a delicate balance between pH levels and beneficial bacteria.

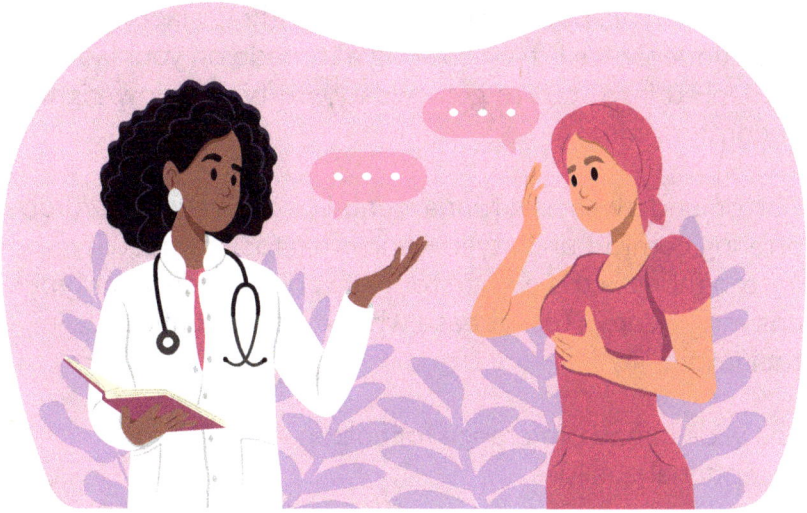

Sarah stared at her underwear drawer with a newfound sense of purpose. After her rather enlightening trip to the gynecologist, she wasn't taking any chances with her vaginal health. It was time to bid farewell to those lacy numbers and embrace the almighty power of cotton.

Now, why is there all the fuss about cotton underwear? Well, let me break it down for you. Cotton is like the superhero of fabrics regarding your lady bits. It's breathable, absorbent, and oh-so-comfortable - everything you want in a pair of panties.

Cotton Only, Please: Why Lace Might Be Pretty, But Cotton Is Queen When It Comes To Your Panties

Your vagina is like a delicate flower garden, and cotton underwear is the gentle breeze that keeps everything fresh and flourishing. But toss in a pair of synthetic, lacey undies, and suddenly, it's like unleashing a tornado on your lady garden - things start to get sweaty, stuffy, and downright uncomfortable.

Cotton underwear is a fundamental piece in every wardrobe, offering comfort and style. Renowned for its versatility, cotton fabric is the cornerstone of various underwear types, ensuring wearers feel at ease while exuding confidence in their attire.

The widespread preference for cotton stems from its exceptional qualities:

First and foremost, cotton reigns supreme in breathability among all fabrics. As a natural fiber, it can whisk away moisture, allowing the body to remain cool and fresh even during scorching temperatures. Unlike synthetic materials prone to trapping bacteria and causing unpleasant odors, cotton fosters healthier skin by maintaining a breathable environment.

Furthermore, cotton boasts unparalleled softness, providing a luxurious feel against the skin. Unlike its synthetic counterparts, which may cause discomfort and irritation due to heat retention and friction, cotton's inherent elasticity ensures a snug yet comfortable fit. Opting for loose-fitting underwear with a gentle elastic waistband prevents chafing and promotes overall comfort throughout the day.

Durability is another hallmark of cotton underwear. Resistant to shrinkage and fading, cotton garments retain their shape and color even after multiple washes. Machine washable and tumble-dry safe, they offer convenience without compromising quality. However, proper care is essential to preserve their softness and longevity. Washing in cold water and air drying helps maintain their elasticity, especially in humid climates, thus extending their lifespan.

Moreover, cotton underwear transcends mere functionality to embrace fashion-forward designs. Gone are the days of mundane styles, as contemporary options cater to diverse preferences, ranging from minimalist to intricate designs that complement modern fashion trends.

Cotton underwear epitomizes the perfect blend of comfort, durability, and style, making it an indispensable staple in every wardrobe. So, do yourself a favor and swap out those frilly, fancy panties for soft, breathable cotton. Your lady bits will thank you for it, trust me.

Say No To Thongs And Hot Tubs: Examining The Hazards Of Tight Clothing And Frequent Hot Tub Use On Vaginal Health

Picture this: you're getting ready for a night out, slipping into your favorite pair of tight jeans or that cute little thong you've been saving for a special occasion. Sure, they might look great on the outside, but what's going on inside your lady bits?

Tight clothing, especially thongs, might seem like harmless fashion choices, but when it comes to your vaginal health, they can be downright hazardous. Let me break it down for you:

- **Friction and Irritation:** Tight clothing, including thongs, can create friction against your delicate skin, leading to irritation, chafing, and even microtears. Ouch! And let's be real - nobody wants to deal with discomfort down there, especially when you're trying to strut your stuff on the dance floor.

- **Moisture and Heat:** Ever notice how things can get steamy down there, especially on a hot day or after a workout? Well, tight clothing only exacerbates the problem by trapping moisture and heat, creating the perfect breeding ground for bacteria and yeast. Before you know it, you're dealing with a full-blown yeast infection or bacterial overgrowth, and that's not exactly the kind of party you were hoping for.

But wait, it gets even steamier - let's talk about hot tubs. Sure, they might seem like the ultimate relaxation zone, but for your vagina, they're a hotbed of danger. Here's why:

- **Disruption of pH Balance:** Hot tubs are filled with warm, bubbly water, which might feel soothing on the skin but can wreak havoc on your delicate vaginal pH balance. When your pH gets thrown out of whack, it creates the perfect environment for infections to flourish, leaving you vulnerable to discomfort and irritation.

- **Increased Risk of Infections:** Thanks to the warm, moist environment, hot tubs are teeming with bacteria and other microorganisms. When you immerse yourself in that bacteria-infested water, you're essentially inviting trouble into your lady bits. The risks are real, my friend, from urinary tract infections to yeast infections.

So, what's a girl to do? Fear not, for I come bearing practical tips to help you navigate these hazards and protect your precious vaginal health:

- **Opt for Breathable Fabrics:** Say goodbye to tight jeans and hello to loose, breathable fabrics like cotton. Your lady bits will thank you for the extra room to breathe and move freely.

- **Choose underwear Wisely:** When it comes to panties, ditch the thongs and opt for full-coverage styles made of breathable materials. Trust me, your vagina will appreciate the extra support and protection.

- **Limit Hot Tub Time:** While it might be tempting to soak in the warm, bubbly waters of a hot tub, try to limit your time spent soaking to avoid disrupting your vaginal pH balance. Always shower afterward to rinse away any lingering bacteria.

By understanding the risks associated with tight clothing and frequent hot tub use, you can make informed decisions to protect your vaginal well-being. So, think twice next time you're tempted to squeeze into those skinny jeans or dip in the hot tub. Your lady bits will thank you for it, I promise.

♂

Essential Guidelines For Maintaining Vaginal Health Through Underwear Choices

- **Ensure Freshness:** Make it a habit to switch out your underwear daily, and feel free to change more frequently if needed. While conventionally, we wear a single pair per day before tossing it into the laundry, this practice may not always be obligatory. Some medical experts suggest that wearing the same pair for two consecutive days is acceptable, provided there isn't significant discharge or perspiration. However, if you begin to feel discomfort due to an accumulation of vaginal discharge, it's perfectly fine to swap them out more frequently.

- **Embrace Panty-Free Nights:** Whether to sleep sans underwear sparks varied opinions. For individuals with a healthy vaginal ecosystem, either choice is acceptable. However, going underwear-free at bedtime can yield significant benefits for those prone to recurrent yeast infections. Opting out of undergarments allows the area to breathe throughout the night, preventing moisture buildup and the creation of a conducive environment for bacterial growth. If sleeping commando doesn't appeal to you, consider donning loose-fitting pajama bottoms instead. Just remember, if you're skipping underwear but electing other bottom wear, ensure they're washed regularly.

- **Renew Your Underwear Annually:** While it may seem excessive to replace your underwear yearly, it's a practice backed by certain considerations. Despite regular washing, even ostensibly clean underwear can harbor an astonishing amount of bacteria, with reports indicating up to 10,000 living bacteria per garment. This is partly due to bacteria in washing machine water, which can contain millions of bacteria in just a small volume. Additionally, studies have revealed the potential presence of fecal matter in underwear, with an average of about one-tenth of a gram per pair. While discarding underwear annually may not align with eco-conscious ideals, it's worth considering, especially if you experience frequent bacterial vaginosis or related symptoms. Adopting these simple underwear rules can contribute significantly to maintaining optimal vaginal health and overall well-being.

Fragrant Soaps, Yogurt, And Dryer Sheets, Oh My: Uncovering The Surprising Culprits That Could Be Disrupting Your Delicate Balance Down There

Let's start with fragrant soaps and detergents. While they may leave you feeling squeaky clean and smelling like a field of flowers, they often contain harsh chemicals and fragrances that can disrupt the delicate balance of your vaginal microbiome. You see, your vagina is home to a diverse community of bacteria and yeast that work together to maintain optimal health. Introducing harsh chemicals and fragrances into the mix upsets this delicate balance, leading to irritation, itching, and even infections.

However, it's not just soaps and detergents that you need to watch out for. Scented hygiene products, like feminine wipes and sprays, can also wreak havoc on your vaginal health. These products often contain ingredients that can irritate the delicate tissues of the vagina, leading to inflammation and discomfort. Plus, they can throw off the natural pH balance of your vagina, making it more susceptible to infections.

And then there's yogurt. Yes, you read that right - yogurt. While it may be touted as a miracle cure for everything from digestive issues to yeast infections, slathering it on your vagina is not the way to go. It can do more harm than good. Yogurt contains live bacteria cultures, which may sound like a good thing. Still, when introduced into the vagina, they can disrupt the natural balance of bacteria and yeast, leading to infections and irritation.

Last but not least, let's talk about dryer sheets. While they may leave your laundry smelling fresh and clean, they often contain chemicals and fragrances that can transfer onto your underwear. When these chemicals come into contact with the delicate tissues of the vagina, they can cause irritation and inflammation, making you more prone to infections.

So, what's a girl to do? First and foremost, opt for gentle, fragrance-free products specifically designed for use on your lady bits. Look for products that are pH-balanced and free from harsh chemicals and fragrances. Additionally, regularly refresh your panty drawer with soft, breathable cotton underwear. By taking these simple steps, you can promote optimal vaginal hygiene and keep 'Her' happy and healthy.

And there you have it, ladies - a comprehensive look at the surprising culprits that could be disrupting your delicate balance down there. From fragrant soaps and detergents to scented hygiene products and certain foods, it's important to be mindful of what you're putting in and on your body.

3

The Vagina: More Than Just A Pretty Flower

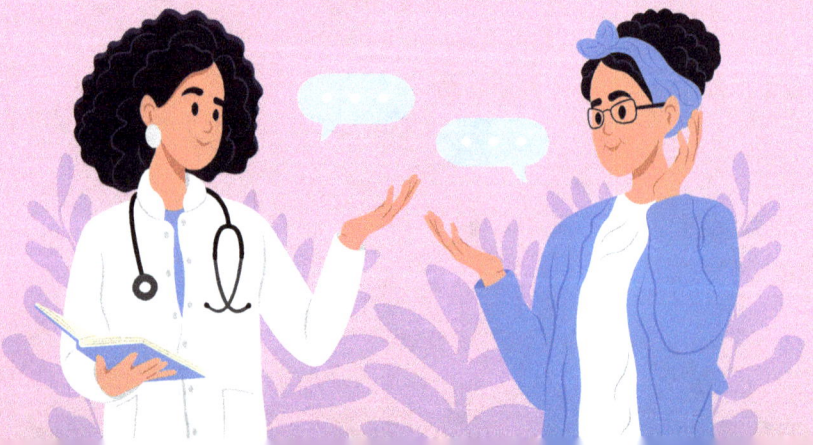

*I*n the last chapter in which we have expounded on the significance of maintaining vaginal health, from understanding pH levels to navigating through the perils of scented soaps as well as thong underwear. Now brace yourself for a deeper plunge into the magical realm that is a vagina where we will cover its anatomy, interpret vaginal discharges and further enter into the age-old discussion on pubic hair politics.

Imagine, you are sitting in your favorite chair sipping tea when out of nowhere someone mentions vaginas. You can actually see everyone leaning closer to learn more about it, ready with curiosity almost palpable in their eyes. After all, you must agree that there is something fresh and thrilling about female reproductive system.

Cheer up readers! This journey is unlike any other. It is an adventure exploring everything from vaginal anatomy's intricacies to discarding mysteries regarding vaginal discharge then cleaning through pubic hair politics' murky waters, enough excitement within Vagina's wild world.

So whether you're a seasoned explorer of the nether regions or just starting off with some curiosity, this chapter has got something for everybody. So put on your safari hat, grab your magnifying glass; it's time to jump right into "The Vagina: More Than Just a Pretty Flower." Trust me; you won't regret it!

Female Reproductive Anatomy Unveiled

Female reproductive organs produce and provide maintenance for female sex cells (eggs or ova), which are conveyed to a place where they can be fertilized by sperm, create an environment favorable to the growth of the fetus, move the fetus outwards at the end of its development period and secrete the female sex hormones. The woman's reproductive mechanisms include: ovaries, fallopian tubes, uterus, vagina, accessory glands as well as external genitalia.

- **Ovaries:**

  Our first stop is ovaries – which are the main organs that manufacture eggs ova as well as secreting hormones necessary for reproduction. These almond-shaped powerhouses reside in pelvic cavities producing eggs nonstop throughout a process known as ovulation. Each ovary is a solid ovoid structure about 3.5 cm long, 2 cm wide and 1 cm thick—that is roughly the size and shape of an almond nut. They are located in shallow depressions known as ovarian fossae situated with one on each side of uterus in the lateral walls of pelvis cavity. Loose peritoneal ligaments hold them in place.

- **Fallopian tube:**

  Moving down the anatomical roadmap, we encounter the fallopian tubes, delicate structures resembling slender tubes adorned with delicate fimbriae at their distal ends.

These fallopian tubes serve as the conduits through which eggs travel from the ovaries to the uterus, where the magic of fertilization awaits. In essence, these are narrow tubes that are attached to the upper part of your uterus and serve as pathways for your egg (ovum) to travel from your ovaries to your uterus. Fertilization of an egg by sperm normally occurs in the fallopian tubes. The fertilized egg then moves to the uterus, where it implants into your uterine lining.

- **Uterus:**

Then, we arrive at the pièce de résistance – the uterus. This pear-shaped organ, with its muscular walls and intricate architecture, serves as the nurturing cradle for developing embryos. During menstruation, the inner lining of the uterus, known as the endometrium, sheds in preparation for potential implantation. If fertilization occurs, the embryo implants itself into the endometrial lining, initiating the journey of pregnancy.

Even so, our anatomical expedition does not end there. Now, we must also pay homage to the vagina, the gateway to the reproductive kingdom. This elastic canal, with its remarkable ability to stretch and accommodate, serves as the passageway for menstrual flow, sexual intercourse, and childbirth. Lined with mucous membranes and guarded by a complex ecosystem of bacteria, the vagina plays a crucial role in maintaining vaginal health and protecting against infections

- **External Parts:**

  Shall we talk about those external genitals? Their job is like a bouncer at a club - keeping everything safe from intruders while allowing the VIPs (sperm) to make their grand entrance into the party (your vagina).

First off, meet your vulva - the superstar collective of all things external down there. People often mix it up and call everything the vagina, but nope, your vagina is its own cozy space inside your body, like a secret hideout for special occasions.

Now, onto the main attractions:

- **Labia Majora:** Think of these as the bodyguards, enclosing and safeguarding the rest of the gang. Oh, and during puberty, they get a stylish makeover with some hair and their very own sweat and oil glands - talk about glam!

- **Labia Minora:** These are the petite pals nestled inside the labia majora, framing the entrances to both the magical land of menstruation (your vagina) and the pee parade (your urethra). Handle with care - they're delicate flowers prone to puffing up if not treated gently.

- **Clitoris:** The star of the show! Your personal pleasure button, tucked away but not forgotten. It's like the mini version of a penis, with its very own hood for protection. Handle with care and be prepared for fireworks.

- **Vaginal Opening:** The grand exit for all things menstrual and baby-related. But hey, it's also the entrance for tampons, fingers, toys, or the occasional adventurous penis - variety is the spice of life, right?

- **Hymen:** The mysterious piece of tissue that gets everyone talking. It's like nature's little curtain, present during birth and often making headlines.

- **Opening to Your Urethra:** Last but not least, the pee portal. It's small but mighty, handling its business like a champ.

—————— ♂ ——————

Well, there you have it, your very own girl squad downstairs, keeping things interesting and occasionally surprising. Embrace the uniqueness, ladies!

As we reflect on the intricate interplay of organs within the female reproductive system, we are reminded of the awe-inspiring complexity of life itself. From the rhythmic dance of hormones to the seamless orchestration of ovulation and menstruation, every aspect of the female anatomy is a testament to the beauty and resilience of the human body.

Howbeit, beyond the realm of biology lies a deeper message - one of empowerment and appreciation for the miraculous capabilities of the female body. In embracing the intricacies of our anatomy, we reclaim ownership of our reproductive health and celebrate the inherent strength and beauty of womanhood.

Vaginal Discharge

Vaginal complaints account for approximately 10 million primary care visits annually in the United States alone. It is the most common gynecological complaint seen by primary care doctors, yet rates of misdiagnosis are high. Vaginal discharge may be a normal physiologic occurrence or a pathological manifestation. It's a topic that often elicits discomfort and uncertainty, yet holds the key to understanding our vaginal health like never before. Let's embark on a journey through the labyrinth of discharge, decoding its mysteries and uncovering the truths hidden within.

Vaginal discharge is a natural and normal occurrence, serving as the body's way of maintaining vaginal health and cleanliness. It's like Mother Nature's very own self cleaning mechanism, flushing out bacteria, dead cells, and other debris to keep the vagina in tip-top shape. Nevertheless, exactly what constitutes "normal" discharge, and when should you be concerned?

Normal vaginal discharge can vary in color, consistency, and odor throughout the menstrual cycle. At its most basic level, it's typically clear or milky-white, with a slight odor that is not unpleasant. However, factors such as hormonal fluctuations, sexual arousal, and even diet can influence the characteristics of discharge. But fear not! Healthy discharge doesn't come with a side of itching, redness, or swelling, and it certainly doesn't have a scent that could knock out a room. It's just your body doing its thing, especially when your estrogen levels are having a party during ovulation, puberty, or pregnancy. So, if you're in the 10% club of those with normal vaginal discharge, congratulations – your vagina is basically winning at life!

On the flip side, abnormal discharge may signal an underlying issue that requires attention. Changes in color (such as yellow, green, or gray), consistency (becoming thicker or clumpy), or odor (strong, fishy, or foul-smelling) may indicate infection or inflammation. Additionally, accompanying symptoms like itching, burning, or irritation further suggest an imbalance in vaginal health.

If your discharge decides to change its color, consistency, volume, or aroma, and brings along symptoms like itchiness, soreness, or pelvic pain, well, that's when things get interesting. It's like your vagina's way of saying, "Plot twist!" So, if you're experiencing intermenstrual bleeding or postcoital bleeding, it might be time to have a chat with your gynecologist. And here's a pro tip: if your discharge starts acting like a diva – significantly altering its usual pattern, showing up with a new color palette, or even throwing in some blood – it's less likely to be just a part of the natural flow. Time to hit the brakes and seek some professional advice. Your vagina will thank you later!

Understanding the nuances of vaginal discharge is crucial for recognizing when something may be amiss and seeking appropriate medical care. Whether it's a yeast infection, bacterial vaginosis, or sexually transmitted infection, early detection and treatment are key to preventing complications and restoring vaginal health.

In essence, vaginal discharge is more than just a bodily fluid - it's a barometer of vaginal health, a testament to the body's innate wisdom, and a call to action for self-care and empowerment. So, let's embrace the complexities of discharge, decode its messages, and celebrate the marvels of the vagina in all its glory.

Pubic Hair Politics

The hairy world of pubic hair politics – a topic that has sparked debates and discussions in bedrooms, boardrooms, and beauty salons alike. Let's dive into this tangled web of personal grooming choices and explore the implications for vaginal health and societal norms.

In recent years, pubic hair grooming trends have shifted dramatically. Gone are the days when a full bush was the norm; instead, we're faced with a plethora of options, from full Brazilian waxes to neatly trimmed landing strips and everything in between. But what impact do these grooming practices have on vaginal health?

Some argue that going au naturel is the best option, as pubic hair serves as a natural barrier, protecting the delicate skin of the genital area from friction and irritation. Plus, it's been suggested that pubic hair may play a role in trapping pheromones, the chemical signals that help attract potential mates. In this sense, pubic hair could be seen as a biological advertisement for sexual readiness.

On the other hand, proponents of hair removal argue that keeping things trimmed and tidy can improve hygiene and reduce the risk of bacterial and fungal infections. They also point to cultural and societal pressures, with many viewing hairless genitals as more aesthetically pleasing or sexually desirable.

But here's the thing – there's no one-size-fits-all answer when it comes to pubic hair grooming. What works for one person may not work for another, and that's okay. The key is to find a grooming routine that makes you feel comfortable, confident, and, most importantly, healthy.

──────────── ♂ ────────────

With that being said, it's essential to approach pubic hair grooming with caution. Shaving, waxing, and other hair removal methods can cause skin irritation, ingrown hairs, and even infections if not done properly. Plus, overzealous grooming practices can disrupt the delicate balance of bacteria and yeast in the genital area, leading to unpleasant odors, itching, and discomfort.

Whether you choose to rock a full bush, keep things neatly trimmed, or go completely bare down there, the most important thing is to prioritize your vaginal health. Listen to your body, pay attention to any signs of irritation or discomfort, and don't be afraid to switch up your grooming routine if something isn't working for you.

At the end of the day, pubic hair politics is about more than just personal preference – it's about embracing diversity, challenging societal norms, and empowering individuals to make informed choices about their bodies. So, let's celebrate the beauty and uniqueness of every pubic hair, regardless of how it's styled. After all, when it comes to pubic hair politics, there's no right or wrong answer – just a whole lot of hair-raising discussions!

Well, folks, we've certainly taken quite the journey through the wonderful world of the vagina, haven't we? From dissecting its anatomy to decoding the mysteries of vaginal discharge and navigating the treacherous terrain of pubic hair politics, we've covered it all – and then some.

However, before we bid adieu to our lady bits for now, let's take a moment to reflect on all we've learned. After all, let's face it – who knew that the humble vagina could be such a source of fascination and amusement?

So, whether you're feeling inspired to give your pubic hair a makeover or you're just grateful to know the difference between normal discharge and something worth calling your gynecologist about, one thing's for sure: your vagina is one heck of a complex, beautiful, and endlessly fascinating organ.

4

Periods: The Monthly Visitor

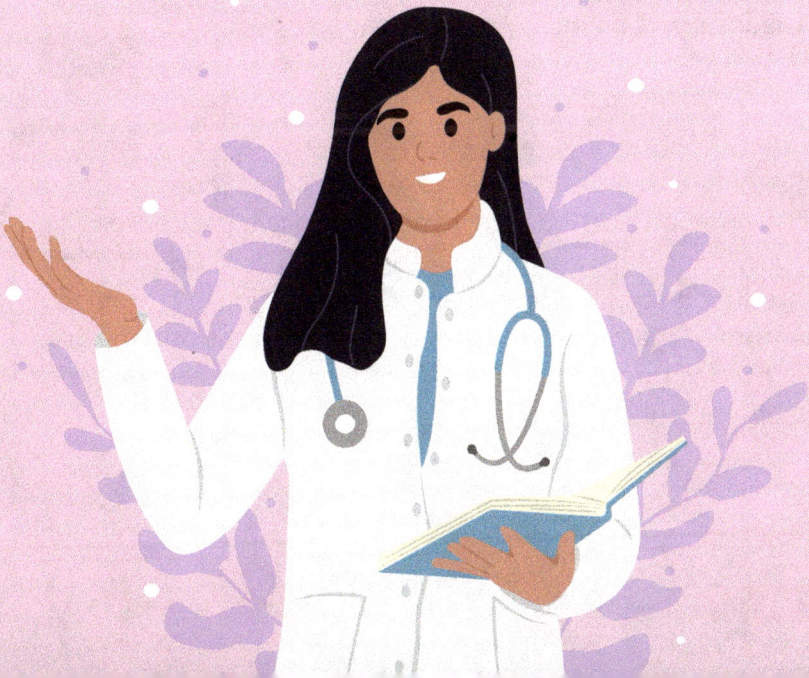

*I*n the last chapter, we've explored the wonders of vaginal anatomy, decoded the mysteries of vaginal discharge, and even tackled the hairy world of pubic hair politics. Now, get ready to dive into the tumultuous waters of menstruation, where Aunt Flo pays her monthly visit, PMS wreaks havoc, and sustainable period products offer a glimmer of hope in the chaos.

But fear not, brave souls, for we are not merely spectators in this monthly spectacle – we are warriors, armed with laughter, empathy, and a dash of chocolate for good measure. So let's cast aside the stigma, break free from the shackles of silence, and boldly confront the taboo that surrounds menstruation.

In this chapter, we'll take a lighthearted look at Aunt Flo's grand entrance, offering a humorous perspective on the joys and challenges of menstruation. From the quirks of PMS to the triumphs of sustainable period products, we'll explore every twist and turn of the menstrual cycle with wit, wisdom, and a healthy dose of sarcasm.

───────── ♂ ─────────

So join us, dear readers, as we embark on a journey through the crimson tide – where every cramp is a battle won, every chocolate craving a victory dance, and every period product a step towards menstrual liberation. It's time to embrace the monthly visitor with open arms and a sense of humor, for in the world of "Periods: The Monthly Visitor," laughter truly is the best medicine.

Aunt Flo's Arrival

Welcome to the monthly spectacle, where Aunt Flo makes her grand entrance, bringing with her a whirlwind of emotions, bodily changes, and a rollercoaster ride of experiences.

The delightful monthly ritual we fondly call menstruation. It's like a surprise party your uterus throws every month, complete with confetti made of tissue and blood. You might also know it as your "time of the month," "Aunt Flo's visit," or simply "that thing I wish I could skip."

So, here's the lowdown: Your body's hormones are the puppet masters behind this whole show. They're like the backstage crew pulling the strings, making sure everything runs smoothly (or not so smoothly, depending on the month). Your brain's pituitary gland and your ovaries team up to produce these hormone maestros, orchestrating a symphony of changes throughout your cycle.

Your uterus, the ever hopeful optimist, decides to spruce things up each month, just in case a tiny tenant decides to move in. It fluffs up its lining, rolls out the welcome mat, and eagerly awaits the arrival of an egg. Meanwhile, your ovaries are like, "Hey, here's an egg! Anyone want to dance?" If Mr. Sperm doesn't show up for the party, well, the uterus has to tidy up and start planning for the next potential guest.

And thus, the period. Cue the dramatic exit as your uterus bids farewell to its carefully prepared accommodations, and you're left wondering why your body insists on throwing this monthly shindig.

Phases Of The Menstrual Cycle

Alright, let's take a rollercoaster ride through the phases of your menstrual cycle, shall we?

- **The Menses Phase:** The grand opening! It's like the red carpet event of your uterus, kicking off as soon as your period RSVPs. Cue the shedding of the uterine lining through the VIP exit, aka your vagina. Don't worry if it lasts anywhere from three to seven days; it's just your uterus doing its thing.

- **The Follicular Phase:** Think of this as the pregame before the main event. Estrogen's rising, and your uterus is getting all dressed up with nowhere to go. Meanwhile, the follicle-stimulating hormone (FSH) is playing fairy godmother to those ovarian follicles, making sure they grow up big and strong. By days 10 to 14, it's like a teenage makeover montage as one lucky follicle becomes a mature egg, ready to take on the world.

- **Ovulation:** The climax! Around day 14, the luteinizing hormone (LH) throws the ultimate egg-release party in your ovary. It's like your ovary saying, "Catch me if you can!" as it releases its precious cargo into the wilds of your fallopian tubes.

- **The Luteal Phase:** Now, we enter the waiting game. Your egg is on a quest to find its destiny in your uterus, while progesterone swoops in to spruce up the place, just in case pregnancy decides to drop by. If the egg finds love and decides to stick around, congratulations! If not, it's back to square one as your uterus throws its own little cleanup crew party.

So there you have it, the menstrual cycle: natures very own soap opera, complete with drama, suspense, and a whole lot of hormones calling the shots.

Women usually start noticing physical and mood changes about 1-2 weeks before period bleeding starts. Changing hormones are to blame for many uncomfortable or unpleasant period signs and symptoms like cramps and tender breasts. Brain chemicals are also involved, but it's unclear to what extent. Period signs and symptoms usually end about 3- 4 days after bleeding begins.

Common signs that your period is approaching are:

To begin with, we should consider the physical symptoms. For many people the onset of menstruation is marked by cramps-those troublesome and sometimes disabling stomach aches that go along with shedding of the lining of the uterus. However, there is no need to fret because there are many strategies that can help you when it comes to this tough path. This may be in terms of heating pads or over-the-counter pain relievers; finding these effective coping mechanisms will go a long way in alleviating discomfort and making you feel lighter during your period.

However, cramps are only the tip of the iceberg. A number of women suffer from bloating when they have their periods and it makes them feel swollen as well as uncomfortable. This may be worsened by hormonal changes and fluid retention causing a feeling of heaviness as well as weariness. Nonetheless, staying hydrated, eating balanced meals and including gentle exercises in your daily routine can aid in reducing bloating hence making one look more normal.

Meanwhile, we could never talk about menstruation without talking about mood swings, for sure! The roller coaster of PMS (premenstrual syndrome) which ranges from inexplicable bouts of sadness to sudden bursts of irritability affects so many individuals. Instead of seeing these frequent mood swings as a burden though, maybe we can think about them differently so that they become our self-care reminders, lessons that teach us how important our mental wellbeing is before anything else. Staying calm by taking a relaxing bath perhaps, engaging in some activities that bring joy or allowing oneself to experience whatever emotions flow freely can be great methods to help deal with PMS; therefore, improving Aunt Flo's stay.

Also, what would Aunt Flo's visit be without cravings? Oh my! The dietary desires associated with menses are downright epic: whether it is an out-of-nowhere yen for chocolate or craving salty snacks or even having an irresistible desire for carbohydrates. However, don't rush towards the nearest tub of ice-cream; instead, consider eating a healthy and well-balanced meal that will help stabilize your blood sugar levels hence, reducing your cravings as much as possible.

Other signs include:

- **Acne Attack:** Yep, your face might decide to throw a party right before your period. It's like your hormones are having their own version of Coachella. Blame those pesky hormones for inviting pimples to the party, especially around your chin and jawline. It's called cyclical acne because, well, it's got its own calendar.

- **Boob Woes:** The joys of tender ta-tas. Thanks to the hormone brigade, your breasts might feel like they've been bench-pressing emotions all month. Cyclical breast pain is the culprit, making your twins feel like they're auditioning for a part in a melodrama.

- **Sleepy Hollow:** Are hormones playing tag with your sleep? Welcome to the club! They love to mess with your internal clock, leaving you feeling like you've been hit by a sleepy truck. Blame estrogen and progesterone for turning your bed into a battleground.

- **The Digestive Tango:** Constipation or diarrhea, anyone? Your digestive system decides to join the pre-period party by doing the cha-cha of extremes. It's like your gut can't decide whether it wants to hold onto everything or let it all go.

- **Bloat City:** It's like your body decided to store up for a rainy day, leaving you feeling like a puffy marshmallow; but fear not, you can fight back with a salt-free diet, veggies for days, and a little dance with the treadmill.

- **Headache Highway:** If your head starts pounding, blame it on the hormonal highway. Estrogen levels are playing bumper cars with your brain, especially if you're prone to migraines. It's as if your period decided to throw in a bonus round of pain, just for fun.

- **Back Attack:** Who knew period cramps had a backstage pass to your lower back? Those sneaky prostaglandins are pulling double duty, causing contractions not just in your belly, but in your back and thighs too. It's like a full-body workout, minus the gym membership.

In addition to these physical and emotional symptoms, menstruation also presents logistical challenges that must be navigated with grace and humor. From discreetly carrying supplies to dealing with unexpected leaks, finding strategies to manage the practical aspects of menstruation can help maintain confidence and peace of mind during Aunt Flo's visit.

Overall, while menstruation may come with its fair share of challenges, it's also a powerful reminder of the strength and resilience of the human body. By embracing the regular and familiar signs of menstruation with humor, empathy, and self-care, we can navigate Aunt Flo's arrival with grace and dignity, emerging on the other side with a renewed sense of empowerment and appreciation for the incredible journey of womanhood.

Coping Mechanism

Now you've entered the wonderful world of PMS, where emotions run high and cravings are real. Don't worry, you're not alone on this rollercoaster ride! Statistics say three out of four of us experience it to some degree. Yep, it's like a monthly subscription to mood swings and bloating.

- **Embrace the Era of Apps:**

  Ever wished you had a crystal ball to predict your mood swings? Well, there's an app for that! Cue Clue or Flo, your trusty sidekicks in the battle against PMS. They'll help you track your cycle and maybe even crack a joke or two to lighten the mood.

- **Ride the Emotional Rollercoaster:**

  When PMS hits, don't try to wrestle with your feelings. Let them flow like a river of emotions. Remember, it's temporary like a storm passing through. Just grab your emotional umbrella and ride it out.

- **Exercise:**

  It might sound crazy to hit the gym when all you want to do is curl up with a tub of ice cream but trust me, exercise is your new BFF during PMS. It's like magic, melting away stress and boosting your mood. Just do it, even if you have to drag yourself there kicking and screaming.

- **Food:**

  Say adios to salt, caffeine, and alcohol – they're just troublemakers during PMS. Instead, load up on H2O, swap sugar for sanity, and embrace foods packed with calcium like they're your new BFF.

- **Chillax and De-Stress:**

  Stressed spelled backward is desserts, but indulging in sweets won't fix everything. Try yoga, meditation, or blasting your favorite tunes to calm the chaos inside. And hey, if all else fails, there's always stress-busting activities of a more intimate nature.

- **Sleep Like a Queen:**

  Don't underestimate the power of shut-eye. Eight hours of beauty sleep is your secret weapon against PMS-induced madness. So, snuggle up and let your dreams be your escape from reality.

- **Buddy Up for Sanity:**

  When PMS threatens to turn you into a hormonal Hulk, call in reinforcements. Gather your squad – friends, family, and significant other – and bask in the healing power of laughter and love. They'll be your sanity-saving superheroes.

Remember, PMS might be a monthly nuisance, but with a little humor and self-care, you'll conquer it like the fierce warrior you are!

Tracking Your Period

Do you wish to become an expert in tracking your menstruation? Well strap yourself in, because we are about to take a journey through the enigmatic world of menstrual cycles.

First up, let us discuss why it is important to know when to expect your period. Yes, I know it may not be as interesting as viewing pictures on Instagram but trust me you need it. When one expects her period and does not get it, this might be a signal that something wrong is happening within her body. Furthermore, who wants surprises there?

Moreover, having insight into your cycle can help you make critical decisions. Like did you know that knowing when you ovulate can boost or lower the chances of getting pregnant? This is like having a fertility magic 8 ball.

Now onto the gritty details of tracking your period down. Get a calendar and start putting X's on it like you're planning some covert operation or something. Day one = x bleeding day = x days without bleeding = pen down till she comes again with her grand entrance.

But if all this sounds too tedious for you then don't worry! There are several apps available that will do all the work for you. It is like having a mobile phone with applications capable of doing anything including tracking periods-it's incredible!

Also, couldn't you go beyond just marking out the basics? Be innovative while doing so! Write from flow intensity (because who doesn't love a flow chart?) to mood swings and motivation levels and even moon phrases (just for fun). One might even end up finding out if lunar phases cause PMS rage.

Besides, the more detailed your charting is, the more ninjy-ish one feels about reporting their periods each month. So step up to the data my friend and come with me into this abyss called menstrual mysteries!

────────────── ♂ ──────────────

Sustainable Period Products

As the world is becoming more eco-conscious, it's not a surprise that sustainable period products are gaining popularity among menstruators. The days when people solely relied on disposable pads and tampons are gone – now menstrual cups, reusable cloth pads and period underwear have gained pace as earth-friendly alternatives; but what exactly are sustainable period products and why should you consider changing to them?

Let us first delve into the world of menstrual cups. These are bell-shaped devices made from medical-grade silicone or rubber which collect menstrual blood rather than absorb it. Menstrual cups can be used over several years, apart from reducing waste generation by disposable pads and tampons. Moreover, they save money for women in terms of monthly period supplies thus being more economical.

The next items are reusable cloth pads. These sort of pads look like their throw-away counterparts but use fabrics like cotton or bamboo to siphon away flows throughout menstruation cycles. After using these cloth pads, one can wash them instead of using single-use ones that add up to landfill waste. Reusable cloth pads exist in different forms including absorbencies so all types of menstruators will find what they need.

Lastly, we have period underwear – a game-changer in the world of menstrual hygiene. These special undies have innermost layers designed to soak up moisture and trap blood to keep you dry and comfortable all day long. Period underwear just like reusable cloth pads can be washed and used over and over again thereby leading to reduction in cost with time.

However, there are many other benefits that come with this kind of environmentally friendly sanitary wear as well. To start with, users experience fewer leakages or odors with menstrual cups/cloth pads/period underwear compared to disposable products according to most people who use it during their menses. Additionally, they do not contain harmful chemicals and other additives commonly found in some disposable tampons and sanitary towels making them safer for your body.

———————— ♂ ————————

Nevertheless, it is important to note that not everyone can use sustainable period products. Some menstruators may find menstrual cups uncomfortable or difficult to use, while others may prefer the convenience of disposable pads and tampons. Furthermore, particularly those in resource-limited settings may face difficulties accessing clean water and private areas required for washing reusable items.

To summarize, sustainable period products are a possible answer to environmental worries and health issues connected with conventional sanitary towels. Women changing from disposable pads/tampons into menstrual cups/reusable cloth pads/period underwear will save money, cut down their carbon footprint and have a much easier and chemical-free period experience. However, choosing the right period product starts by considering individual preferences, needs and available resources.

Sexual Health: Getting Busy Down There

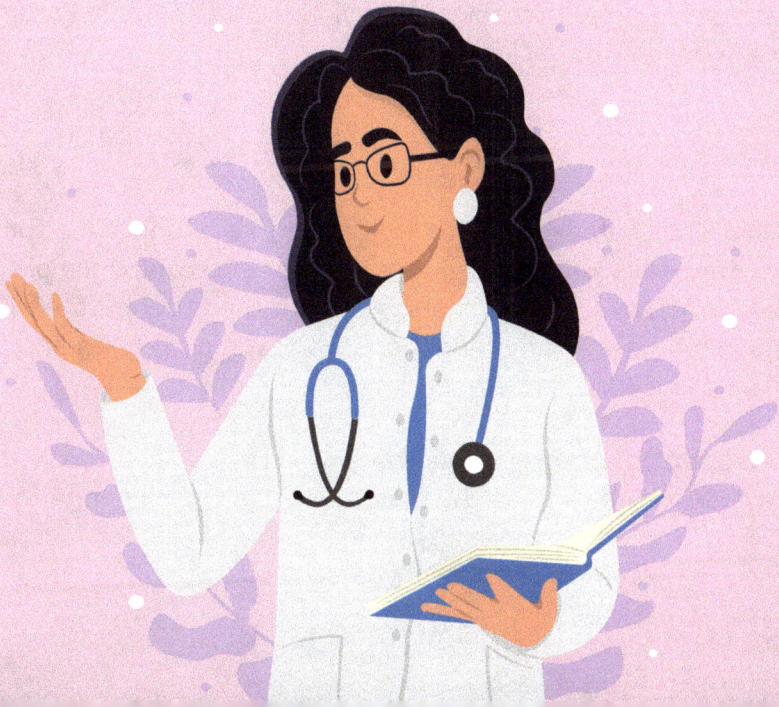

*I*magine you're nestled cozily in bed with your significant other, the air charged with anticipation and desire. But wait, amidst the fervor, a pesky thought creeps in – are we really playing it safe? It's a worry that has haunted many, emphasizing the crucial dance between pleasure and precaution in matters of sexual health.

Now, let's dive into the realm of sexual health, where pleasure meets prudence, and getting frisky becomes both an art and a science. Amidst the throes of passion, it's easy to forget the importance of safety and proper care. So, how do we navigate this delicate balance with poise and confidence? Buckle up, my friends, as we unravel the mysteries of safe sex, the elusive Big O, and the post-coital rituals that keep our nether regions singing with joy.

So, grab your preferred flavored lube and get ready for a ride filled with giggles, enlightenment, and plenty of steamy moments. It's time to embrace the adventure – safely, sensually, and with a hefty dose of humor. After all, laughter is the best aphrodisiac!

Safe Sex

What does safe sex mean? It is similar to a bubble wrap for your genitalia just making sure that not even an ounce of semen, vaginal fluids or blood gets into the other partner. I mean who wants anything more than awkward stares and pickup lines with cheesy endings?

The opposite of this is unsafe sex whereby you just throw caution to the wind as you play games with your genitals as if they were poker chips in a high stakes game. Who needs safety when they have a chance to roll their dice? Spoiler alert: it usually ends badly.

Oh, and wait for it! Do we know that some sexually transmitted infections like syphilis and genital warts are great party poopers? They move faster than family gossip spreading and leaving you with more regrets than having gotten that bad tattoo while in college.

Even so, there is room for thought about our little angels, isn't it? For instance such unborn children may be infected with congenital syphilis and HIV viruses. What better way to say "hello" into this world apart from getting an STD together with your birth certificate?

Nevertheless fear no more for there is light at the end of all these horrific things. Safe sex keeps one off the STI rollercoaster. So zip it up everyone since no one wants anything that reminds them about those wild days during this ride. Plus souvenirs are not welcome either!

——————— ♂ ———————

Guidelines For Safer Sex

So, you've decided to dive into the thrilling world of safer sex? Congratulations, you're about to embark on an adventure that's slightly less risky than tightrope walking over a pit of hungry crocodiles. Here are some guidelines to ensure your journey is as safe as possible:

- **Monogamy is the Name of the Game:** Stick to one partner like glue, and make sure that partner is also stuck on you like a stubborn piece of gum on the bottom of a shoe. This reduces the chance of playing host to uninvited guests in your nether regions.

- **The Talk Before the Walk:** Before getting down and dirty with someone new, engage in a riveting conversation about past partners, STI history, and recreational drug use. It's like a prelude to the main event, but with more awkwardness.

- **Wrap it Up:** Condoms are your best friend. Opt for latex or polyurethane, unless you're allergic to latex, in which case, go for the polyurethane variety. Remember, while nonoxynol-9 might sound like a superhero spermicide, its effectiveness against HIV is about as clear as mud.

- **Say No to Liquid Courage:** While a few shots of tequila might make you feel invincible, they also increase the likelihood of engaging in risky behavior. So, save the booze for celebrating your newfound commitment to safer sex.

- **Ditch the Douche:** Ladies, resist the urge to douche post-coitus. It's about as effective at preventing STIs as using a feather duster to clean a nuclear fallout zone. Plus, it could just end up spreading unwanted guests further up the reproductive tract.

- **Keep Tabs on Your Bits:** Stay vigilant for any suspicious-looking sores, blisters, rashes, or mysterious discharges on either you or your partner's body. Think of it as a sexy game of spot the difference, but with more medical implications.

- **Get Regular Check-Ups:** Make sure to schedule your Pap tests, pelvic exams, and STI screenings like clockwork. It's like maintaining your car, except instead of changing the oil, you're checking for signs of impending sexual doom.

- **Think Outside the Bedroom:** Get creative with your sexual repertoire and explore activities that don't involve fluid exchange or membrane-to-membrane contact. After all, who says you can't have fun without risking your health?

So there you have it, folks. Follow these guidelines, and you'll be navigating the choppy waters of safer sex like a seasoned captain of the SS Responsibility.

Condoms

Condoms – the unsung heroes of safe escapades. They're not just your average latex pouches; they come in all sizes, colors, and even flavors (yes, you read that right). They're like the Swiss Army knives of the bedroom, protecting you from those unexpected surprises. Whether you're flying solo or engaging in some hot partner action, condoms are your trusty sidekick in the battle against STIs like chlamydia, gonorrhea, and the dreaded "gift that keeps on giving," herpes. When it comes to condoms, it's better to wrap it up than face the consequences.

These nifty devices are your go-to barrier against unwanted guests. Picture them as the bouncers at the club, ensuring only the right stuff gets through. We've got a variety to choose from:

- **Male (or external) condoms:** These babies are like the knights in shining armor, made of thin, sturdy latex, and they come in all shapes and sizes. (Sorry, no one-size-fits-all here.) For those allergic to latex, fear not, there are non-latex options available.

- **Female (or internal) condoms:** Think of these as the undercover agents of protection. They're a soft pouch made of synthetic rubber, sporting two flexible rings at each end. They're pre-lubricated and ready to slide into action, fitting snugly inside the vagina or anus.

- **Diaphragms:** These are like the stealth mode of contraception, a soft silicone cup that cozies up inside the vagina, guarding the entrance to the uterus like a pro. They're great for preventing pregnancy, but remember, they don't offer protection against STIs.

You can find condoms pretty much everywhere these days - supermarkets, pharmacies, sexual health clinics, and family planning centers. Heck, you can even snag them from vending machines at your local hotspots like nightclubs, pubs, and colleges. So, no excuses, folks! Stay safe out there.

Contraception

Now, let's talk contraception – because let's face it, accidents happen, and we'd rather not have any unexpected visitors crashing the party nine months down the line. Contraception is defined as the intentional prevention of conception through the use of various devices, sexual practices, chemicals, drugs, or surgical procedures. Thus, any device or act whose purpose is to prevent a woman from becoming pregnant can be considered contraception. In any social context effective contraception allows a couple to enjoy a physical relationship without fear of an unwanted pregnancy and ensures enough freedom to have children when desired. The aim is to achieve this with maximum comfort and privacy, minimal cost and side effects. Some barrier methods, like male and female condoms, also provide the twin advantage of protection from sexually transmitted diseases (STDs).

From the pill to the patch, the ring to the implant, there are more contraception options out there than flavors at an ice cream parlor. Please remember, contraception isn't just about preventing pregnancy – it's also about protecting yourself from STIs. So, don't forget to double up with condoms for extra peace of mind.

—————— ♂ ——————

Protecting Yourself Against STIs

Sexually transmitted infections (STIs) are like party crashers at a wild bash—showing up uninvited and causing all sorts of chaos. These pesky bugs can sneak into your system through any form of sexual shindig, whether it's a mouth-to-mouth, backdoor boogie, or the good ol' in-and-out. They're also known as sexually transmitted diseases (STDs), giving them that extra ominous vibe.

Now, these STIs come in a variety pack, each with its own set of party tricks. The classics? Burning sensations, itching fits, or unexpected discharges in your nether regions. Here's the kicker—some of these troublemakers don't even bother announcing their presence with symptoms. Sneaky, right?

Oh, and here's the real kicker: STIs are like gossip at a high school reunion—super contagious. You could be hosting a whole STI fiesta without even realizing it. For this reason, the Centers for Disease Control and Prevention (CDC) suggests getting yourself checked regularly if you're an active participant in the dance of love.

STIs shouldn't be taken lightly; they're no joke. Some, like the notorious human immunodeficiency virus (HIV), don't have a cure and can really rain on your parade without proper treatment.

Now, onto the symptoms—think of them as warning signs that your body is not okay with the party crashers. You might spot some unexpected guests like bumps, sores, or warts in places you'd rather not have them. And that's not all—swelling, itching, funky discharge, or even unexpected bleeding could also make an appearance. It's like a bad party playlist, but with bodily discomfort.

Wait, there's more! Your body might start throwing a tantrum, complete with a skin rash, weight loss, or bathroom-related drama. It's your body's way of saying, "Get these gatecrashers outta here!"

So, if you suspect these uninvited guests have crashed your party, it's time for a visit to the doc. They'll give you the lowdown after a thorough inspection and maybe a few tests. And hey, honesty is key here—so spill the beans about your symptoms and your partying history. After a positive diagnosis, it's important to let your partners know so they can get checked too. It might be awkward, but it's better than letting these uninvited guests crash more parties.

Remember, whether you're abstaining, playing it safe with protection, or relying on good condoms, keep your sexual health front and center. It's better to be safe and satisfied than itching and scratching your head in a clinic waiting room, wondering where it all went wrong.

The Big O

The mystery of the female orgasm, which is a mystical world of its own. Yet, some people feel very uneasy about it, but that's why we are friends. It's time to talk about something that has been hushed and avoided for a long time- sexual wellbeing of women. Girls, you also have questions regarding your sexuality probably like any other lady who dares to reflect on the concept of 'elusive O's.

What is an orgasm? In other words, it's like fireworks happening within your body, pleasure accompanying sex. So imagine this: your heart is pounding; muscles are making merry; brain has secreted hormones with elation akin to striking a jackpot.

So let us demystify some myths right now? The first one being that the Big O does not exist for others apart from the lucky few who have seen it in person or something quite elusive. If you think it can be found in a secret cave somewhere then think again! And guess what else? It must not be just thrusting in and out motion all the time. However several tastes one may get from a box of chocolate are similar to many forms of female orgasms because they vary from one individual to another hence making them unique. No standard method here – might involve light touches on the clit or go old school vagina as well as anal penetration.

So let's stop thinking about an orgasm as a rare unicorn and look at it for what it actually is- natural and pleasurable part of human life. Now let us debunk some common misconceptions, okay?

Here's the scoop: there's not just one flavor of female orgasm. Instead of zeroing in on types, let's broaden our horizon and explore the myriad of ways to reach that peak of pleasure. Our bodies are wired with a bunch of nerve-rich spots, ready to party when stimulated. We're talking about the classics like the clitoris, vagina, cervix, nipples, and even the ol' backdoor, the anus. It's often a combo platter of these hotspots that lights up the fireworks. Do note though that each lady comes with her own personalized treasure map of erogenous zones.

- **The age-old myth:** good sex equals simultaneous fireworks for both partners.

While orgasms are like the cherry on top of the sundae, they're not the whole darn dessert. Sometimes, just sharing that intimate connection with your partner, regardless of the finale, is the real jackpot. Think of orgasms as delightful bonuses, not the main event.

Alright, let's debunk this baby-making myth once and for all. For the dudes, yes, they need to launch their little swimmers to kick start the pregnancy party. However, for the ladies, it's not a prerequisite to hit the high note. Orgasms are like the sprinkle on your cupcake: not necessary, but oh-so-nice. Sure, they're fun, stress-relieving, and downright enjoyable; but if you're putting all your eggs in the orgasm basket, you might find yourself stuck in a rut. Relax, enjoy the ride, and if the Big O happens, fabulous! If not, no biggie. Just keep the vibe chill, the pressure off, and who knows, you might just surprise yourself.

- **There's something wrong with me if I don't orgasm.**

If you cannot or do not orgasm, the most important thing to know is that there is nothing wrong with you. You are no less capable of having a healthy and full sex life.

There is a small group of women who are unable to achieve an orgasm and this can be caused by the following factors:

- Medications such as antidepressants
- A history of trauma
- Changes that occur at different life stages (for example menopause, weight loss or gain, stress at work, etc.)
- Unknown reasons (frustratingly)

The good news is that there are things you can do to try and make having an orgasm easier. The first step is to ask yourself some questions and do some homework to figure out what works for you. We all have our own individual quirks, preferences, and abilities in the bedroom, and that's more than okay. As long as the sex you're having is consensual and safe, you are doing it right.

- **Orgasms feel the same to everyone.**

This common misconception is perpetuated by TV shows and movies. They tend to set unrealistic expectations for orgasms, especially in women.

The psychological experience of an orgasm can vary, depending on factors such as how aroused or excited you are, whether there are any distractions, or how much pressure you feel to reach orgasm. Even though the same thing is happening to your body physically, the way it feels can be different based on all these factors. Orgasms aren't always "fireworks" amazing: it might be something as ordinary as, "oh that felt nice".

The experience differs from woman to woman so when you compare notes with your girlfriends, keep this in mind! No two bodies are the same.

Now that we've dispelled the myths, let's dive into the fun stuff – exploring different techniques for achieving the Big O. Whether you're flying solo or with a partner, there are countless paths to pleasure waiting to be discovered. From the tried-and-true clitoral stimulation to the more adventurous realms of G-spot exploration and erogenous zone mapping, the possibilities are endless. So, grab your favorite vibrator, experiment with different positions, and let your curiosity be your guide as you embark on a journey of self-discovery and sensual exploration.

One of the most beautiful aspects of the female orgasm is its diversity. Just as no two snowflakes are alike, no two orgasms are identical. Each one is a unique expression of pleasure, shaped by individual anatomy, desires, and experiences. Some may be quick and intense, like a bolt of lightning striking the sky, while others may build slowly and steadily, like a gentle rain shower on a summer afternoon. And let's not forget the elusive yet tantalizing phenomenon of multiple orgasms – a feat that some are lucky enough to achieve, while others continue to chase the dream. Let's celebrate the wondrous diversity of the female orgasmic experience and embrace the fact that pleasure comes in many shapes, sizes, and sensations.

───────── ♂ ─────────

Post Sex Care

So, you've just had a wild romp in the sheets, but before you drift off into a blissful slumber, it's time to show your lady bits a little TLC. After all, they've just been through a marathon, and they deserve a medal (or at least a warm washcloth).

First things first, let's talk about the cleanup operation. It's like a crime scene investigation, except instead of blood spatter, you're dealing with bodily fluids. Grab your trusty washcloth and some gentle, fragrance-free soap, and get to work cleaning up any residual mess. Think of it as a post-apocalyptic cleanup crew - except instead of zombies, you're battling against stray bodily fluids and hey, who said post-sex cleanup couldn't be a bonding experience? Teamwork makes the dream work, after all.

Now that you've tackled the cleanup, it's time to address the elephant in the room - urinary tract infections (UTIs). Ah yes, the bane of every post-sex bliss, UTIs are like the unwelcome guests that just won't leave the party; but fear not, dear readers, for we've got some tricks up our sleeves to keep those pesky UTIs at bay. First and foremost, make sure to pee after sex - it's like hitting the reset button on your urinary tract, flushing out any potential bacteria that may have found their way into your urethra. If you're feeling extra fancy, you can even indulge in some cranberry juice or supplements, which are rumored to have UTI-fighting properties. It's like giving your urinary tract a little extra backup - just in case.

But wait, there's more – let's not forget about the importance of rest and relaxation post coitus. After all, sex can be a workout (depending on your preferred positions, of course), and your body deserves some downtime to recover. So snuggle up with your partner, cue up your favorite Netflix show, and bask in the afterglow of a job well done. Of course if you're feeling adventurous, you can always indulge in a little post-coital snack – after all, you've earned it.

In conclusion, after sex care is like the crowning moment of a sundae - it gives you that full feeling and satisfaction. Do not neglect sanitization, ignore the UTI prevention guidelines and most importantly remember to take some time and relax while enjoying the fruits of your labor. You have just been through the amazing and extraordinary sexual health journey -now go forth.

6

Pregnancy And Childbirth: The Ultimate Vaginal Workout

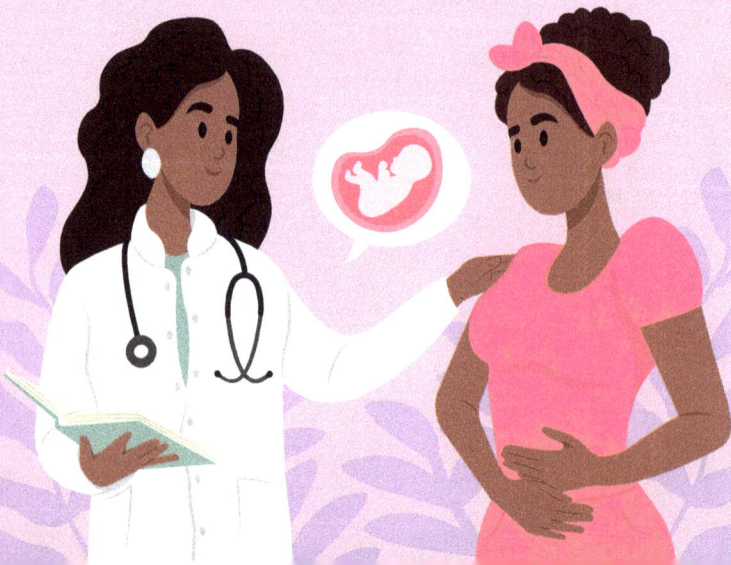

P regnancy – a period during which you may feel amazed, happy, and hungry for some inexplicable peculiar food combinations; but amidst the baby showers and nursery decorating, there's another issue that should draw our attention: how pregnancy affects the vaginal health. Yes, when you are about to start an incredible journey of growing a little human inside your body, it is important to know how this process can influence your vagina wellness.

Suddenly one day in the middle of your second trimester while basking in the glory of motherhood impending; something strange is happening down there! Is it normal? Should I be worried? How do I manage my body changes as well as prepare myself for the delivery?

In this chapter, we will plunge into pregnancy and childbirth – uncovering highs and lows, happiness and problems-from what these hormones mean to the vagina's health during pregnancies to what labor feels like, we shall approach hard questions with laughs, understanding, and empathy. So clutch on to your pregnancy pillow dear one because this journey called pregnancy is about to take you on an adventure that nobody else has ever taken.

Baby On Board: A Journey Through Pregnancy And Its Effect On Vaginal Health

Pregnancy-a jumble of emotions, hunger pains for weird foods, and body transformations that can make even experienced mothers-to-be feel like they're on a roller coaster ride of feelings too hard to control sometimes.

Nevertheless when preparing for their precious bundle of joy women should not fail to observe some bodily changes parting with them mainly being related to vaginal health.

During pregnancy, there are lots of hormonal changes occurring in your body that directly affect your vaginal health. One very noticeable change is increased discharge from the vagina itself. Though it may seem alarming at first sight it is actually normal during pregnancy to have more vaginal discharge because it helps maintain cleanliness in this region. It is usually a thin, milky, white colorless fluid but may take differing consistencies and colors at various stages of pregnancy.

Moreover, hormonal changes that occur during pregnancy may alter the vaginal environment thereby increasing the risk of yeast infections or bacterial vaginosis. The hormone changes provides order to the pH balance of a woman's vagina, making it more susceptible to harmful bacteria or fungi growth. If your vaginal discharge smells bad or is uncomfortable, you should consult a doctor.

Common vaginal infections during pregnancy include:

- **Yeast infections:** During pregnancy, vaginal secretions are sweeter and yeasts feel at home. This infection will not harm your unborn child but it will make you very uncomfortable. Symptoms of yeast infections include vaginal itching, discharge that looks like cottage cheese with a yeasty smell, and painful urination.

- **Bacterial vaginosis (BV):** The American Pregnancy Association states that 10- 30% of pregnant women get bacterial vaginosis. Bacterial imbalances in the vagina cause BV. The main symptom is a gray discharge that smells fishy. If untreated it can lead to premature labor, low birth weight, or miscarriage.

- **Trichomoniasis:** It spreads through sexual contact with an infected person; trichomoniasis may also have severe consequences during pregnancy such as premature rupture of membranes and preterm delivery. The symptoms of trichomoniasis include: yellowish-green discharge with a foul odor, vaginal itching and redness, and pain during sex or while urinating.

And wait for it – let's talk about varicose veins! Yes, you read that right – varicose veins in your lady parts! During pregnancy, vena cava syndrome causes increased pressure on pelvic blood vessels resulting in vulvar or vaginal varicosity development. Though they may be unsightly and uncomfortable they often resolve spontaneously after childbirth although if there is significant pain or discomfort then consult with your healthcare provider about personalized advice and treatment options.

So baby's all cozy while blood runs through your body like a downtown traffic jam at rush hour. Don't be surprised if your lady parts start ballooning up like little balloons. Yeah, well it seems that your labia majora ain't been missing any workouts either! And hey, with all the swelling going on down there too, there might be no stopping your libido from exploding through the roof! Hormones are the culprit here, because now even your private areas could take on weird bluish tones as though you have your discotheque down there.

Now we get to everyone's favorite: vaginal bleeding! The first trimester can be marked with a little bit of light blood flow as the fertilized egg is situated in the uterus. It's almost like your body saying, "Hey I'm just making room for this tiny human, no biggie!" However, if it gets dramatic – think full-on tissue-passing dramatic – you need some help (read: call your doctor). Then zoom forward into later trimesters and out of nowhere comes vaginal bleeding as an unwanted turn of events. We're talking emergency level here - placenta doing the limbo, cervix choosing to host an early party, or even a surprise uterus rupture (yikes!). Now is not the time to release your inner superwoman when something like that happens, let the professionals do their thing.

—————— ♂ ——————

Finally, there is something else you may notice as labor approaches: a bloody show. No, it's not another horror flick; it's just your body preparing for delivery day. One might consider it as a nice invitation sent by your uterus written in pink mucus- RSVP.

Thus, these are some of the unexpected things that come along with pregnancy. Within all the drama unfolding around you remember that your body is quietly performing its miracles. Go ahead and accept being weird and maybe treat yourself with a little more chocolate because why not? You deserve it!

Labor And Delivery

Words cannot truly express the awe-inspiring journey that is childbirth. It is a time of greatest physical endurance for women yet one that showcases their power at its highest limits. But let's be frank here folks; we aren't going to paint rosy pictures. However amazing it might seem, childbirth can be a chaotic and messy experience that leaves even the strongest-willed expectant mothers to question their sanity.

First up: labor pain – because let's face it, they are not exactly walking in the park. The initial labor pains may feel no worse than slight twinges; however, heavy contractions when you think your gut is being punched by an angry mob of kangaroo kickers are nothing to laugh about. And don't worry dear readers we will walk through this chaos full of jokes and ice chips.

Next up, come along as we explore some less glossy truths about delivering a baby vaginally. A process that defies reason; physics and practically every other law of nature that exists. Starting from the primal screams reverberating in the labor room down to the not-so-dainty bodily fluids present during birth, it's a voyage that can test you beyond your physical and emotional boundaries.

But amongst all this disorganization and suffering lies also beauty within the miracle of childbearing. As you hold your infant for the first time, everything around you disappears leaving only that tiny bundle wiggling in your hands making a loud noise on earth. For many people, it is a magical moment whereby they are reminded how powerful human bodies are whilst demonstrating an undying maternal bond.

——————— ♂ ———————

Vaginal Health After Giving Birth

You may have pain coupled with swelling or bruising after any type of vaginal delivery along with pain while urinating or moving your bowels. In most cases, these symptoms get better after a few weeks though they may last longer if your vagina has been torn during childbirth or the skin between your vagina and anus had to be cut to deliver your baby.

Bleeding from the vagina is normal for two to six weeks after delivery. In fact, heavy, bright red bleeding and clots is common for the first day after you have given birth. From this point onwards, it should gradually decrease but you may retain some blood for up to 6 weeks. Your vagina will probably feel wide and stretchy after giving birth. It usually regains much of its elasticity within six weeks. Kegel exercises and other pelvic floor exercises performed during and after pregnancy help increase vaginal tone and decrease your risk of organ prolapse into the vagina.

Women who are breastfeeding have lower estrogen levels and are more likely to experience dryness. Water-based lubricants and natural moisturizers may help relieve vaginal dryness symptoms, such as painful sex, vaginal itching, and vaginal burning. You may find relief from vaginal pain and swelling by doing the following:

- Apply ice packs to the perineal area for the first 24 hours. Ice packs and cold compresses should be removed after 10 to 20 minutes and reapplied every hour as needed. (Ice packs should be wrapped in a towel or facecloth and not applied directly to the skin).

- Women can use cold compresses, a bag of ice or frozen veggies, or a frozen, water soaked maxi-pad or baby diaper to place in their underwear.

- Use a peri-bottle or a spray bottle to rinse off the perineum after using the toilet and blot dry.

  - Rest as much as possible.

  - Let the perineum air-dry while resting.

- Use a pillow or an inflatable ring when sitting. Inflatable rings are available at most drug-stores.

  - Soak the perineal area in warm water a few times a day and after bowel movements. A sit down bath filled with a few inches of water and placed on the toilet seat is convenient and can be purchased at the drugstore or home health store. · If you are using your bathtub for perineal soaks, have it cleaned first and ensure that someone is present to help you in and out of the tub for the first few times. · Take pain medications recommended by your health care provider.

As you prepare to embark on the wild ride that is labor and delivery, remember this: while childbirth may be messy, chaotic, and downright surreal, it's also one of the most profound and awe-inspiring experiences a woman can ever hope to experience.

———————— ♂ ————————

Postpartum Recovery

As you bask in the glow of new motherhood, it's time to turn our attention to the often overlooked phase of postpartum recovery. From stitches to stretch marks, postpartum recovery is a journey of healing, resilience, and self-care – and it's essential to approach it with patience, compassion, and a healthy dose of humor.

Let's start with the basics: postpartum recovery begins the moment your baby is born and continues for weeks, if not months, afterward. During this time, your body undergoes a myriad of changes as it gradually returns to its pre-pregnancy state. One of the most common concerns during this period is healing from any perineal tears or episiotomies that may have occurred during childbirth. These tears, while common, can be painful and require diligent care to ensure proper healing. There are various ways of soothing the pain and ensuring quick healing in this delicate region, from sit baths to witch hazel pads.

Postpartum recovery is not only about physical healing, it also involves emotional and mental health. New moms can be overwhelmed by different emotions during the postnatal stage such as joy for giving birth to a baby, fatigue from night nursing as well as anxiety that comes with having a newborn baby. It is important to prioritize self-care during this period may involve taking deep breaths, asking for help when necessary or getting professional support if you are suffering from postpartum depression/anxiety.

Also, we shouldn't forget about breastfeeding's joys and challenges. Although breastfeeding can be a wonderful way of the mother and child bonding, it could also bring various forms of discomfort including tender nipples, breast fullness engorgement, and mastitis. Proper breastfeeding practices should be learned while assistance from lactation consultants or support groups sought as they can make a huge difference in your own adventure.

Tips To Help Your Postpartum Recovery

Although most of the healing after giving birth happens naturally, there are several things you can do to support your body's recovery.

- **Core muscle workout:** Try exercises that will target the abdominal muscles in your trunk. This will make the muscles strong while giving you more support. ·

- **Prenatal vitamins:** Continue taking prenatal vitamins even as you breastfeed. These will help replace the nutrients lost while pregnant and keep up with your recovery process. The doctor may also advise on some other supplements like iron and vitamin C for added advantages.

- **Kegels or pelvic floor exercises:** After childbirth happens, it is common to have problems with weak pelvic floor muscles (muscles found at the bottom part of the pelvis that offer support to the bladder) which can cause challenges with urination control as well as leaking urine when doing certain activities such as coughing or jumping jacks which causes pressure on those muscles. To avoid this situation consider doing Kegel exercises every day. Do them by squeezing your pelvic floor muscles tight for 3-5 seconds then letting go and repeating.

- **Retinoid creams:** Retinoid creams contain Vitamin A which helps fade stretch marks away from view. The application of some of this cream to one's skin can be advantageous; however, much better if done faster because once they turn white, it could be too late.

- **Sexual intercourse life:** As long as you feel okay about yourself and get a nod from your doctor, go ahead and enjoy sex whenever you desire. Take sex slowly and use vaginal lubricants if necessary.

- **Get Support:** Sometimes when you're a new parent, it feels like everything is on your shoulders but don't be afraid to lean on the family surrounding you when mentally exhausted after childbirth. In many cases, family member's friends or even neighbors are willing to help by allowing you to take a quick nap or walk around the block.

In brief, postpartum recovery is a challenging expedition that necessitates patience, self love, and knowing when to seek assistance. With empathy and light-heartedness, you can navigate postpartum life with all its ups and downs in an elegant way. It is important to remember to remain present, revel in your successes no matter how small they may appear and similarly treat yourself with kindness as you undertake this amazing journey of parenting.

7

Menopause: The Vaginal Saga Continues

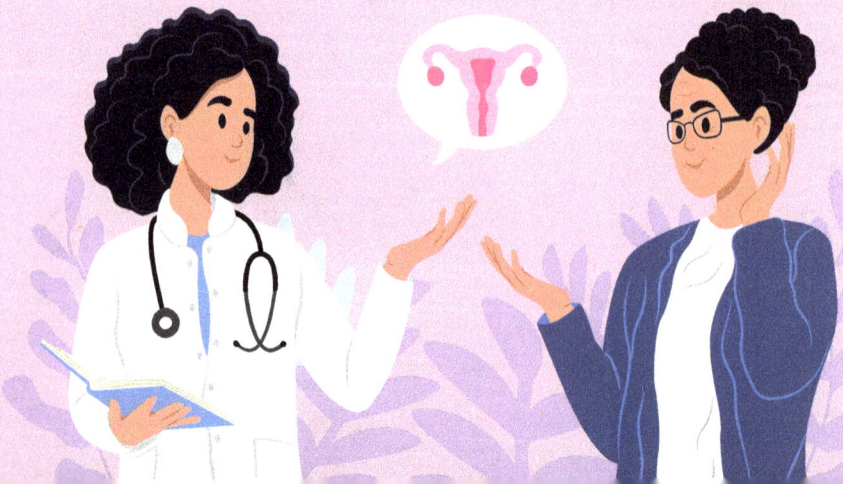

As we embark on this chapter, it's time to grab a cup of tea, cozy up in your favorite chair, and prepare for a candid exploration of the hormonal rollercoaster that is menopause. You're in your fabulous forties or fifties, juggling career, family, and all of life's adventures, when suddenly, you're hit with a wave of hot flashes that could rival the Sahara desert. But fear not, my fellow women, for we are about to delve deep into the mysteries of menopause and its effects on vaginal health.

Menopause isn't just a single event - it's a journey, a transition, and yes, sometimes even a comedy of errors. But amidst the hot flashes and mood swings, there's another aspect of menopause that deserves our attention: its impact on our vaginal well-being.

In this chapter, we'll take a candid look at the hormonal rollercoaster of menopause and how it affects our vaginal health. From the dryness and discomfort that can leave us feeling like a desert oasis to the challenges of navigating intimacy and pleasure during this transformative stage of life, we'll explore it all with humor, insight, and maybe even a few laughs along the way.

So buckle up, because the vaginal saga continues with menopause - but with a bit of humor and a lot of resilience, we can navigate this new chapter with grace and confidence.

Exploring Menopause And Its Effects On Vaginal Health

Let's start with the basics: menopause, that magical time when our estrogen levels take a nosedive, wreaking havoc on everything from our moods to our metabolism – and yes, even our vaginal health. You see, estrogen plays a crucial role in maintaining the thickness and elasticity of vaginal tissues, as well as regulating vaginal moisture levels. So when those estrogen levels plummet, it's like our vaginas are suddenly thrust into a Sahara desert impersonation contest – dry, uncomfortable, and decidedly un-fun.

Wait, there's more! Menopause can also bring about changes in the pH balance of the vagina, creating the perfect breeding ground for pesky infections like yeast and bacterial vaginosis. It's like our vaginas are suddenly hosting a microbial rave – complete with itching, burning, and a general sense of "what the heck is going on down there?" Menopause represents a significant milestone in a person's life, denoting the cessation of menstruation for at least 12 consecutive months. It is a natural phase of aging that signifies the conclusion of one's reproductive years, typically occurring around the age of 51, though individual experiences may vary. Natural menopause, distinct from medically induced menopause, unfolds gradually through three different stages:

- **Perimenopause**

  Perimenopause, often termed the "menopause transition," typically spans eight to 10 years before the onset of menopause, commonly commencing in one's 40s. During this phase, the ovaries gradually reduce estrogen production, leading to irregular menstrual cycles. Perimenopause culminates with menopause, characterized by the cessation of ovulation and menstruation. In the final one to two years of perimenopause, estrogen levels decline more rapidly, accompanied by the onset of menopausal symptoms. Despite experiencing such symptoms, individuals may still conceive during this period.

- **Menopause**

  It signifies the cessation of menstrual periods, indicating that the ovaries have halted egg release and significantly reduced estrogen production. Medical professionals confirm menopause after 12 consecutive months without menstruation.

- **Post menopause**

  It designates the phase following an entire year without menstruation, extending throughout the remainder of one's life. While menopausal symptoms like hot flashes may diminish during this stage, some individuals may continue to experience them for a decade or longer. Postmenopausal individuals face an increased risk of various health conditions, including osteoporosis and heart disease, due to decreased estrogen levels.

Vaginal Dryness And Discomfort

Vaginal dryness often stems from a decrease in estrogen levels, typically occurring as menopause approaches. Estrogen, produced by the ovaries, regulates various female body characteristics and functions, including the thickness and moisture of vaginal tissues. When estrogen levels decline, the vaginal lining may become thinner, drier, and less elastic, a condition known as vaginal atrophy. Factors contributing to reduced estrogen levels include surgical removal of the ovaries, childbirth, breastfeeding, and hormonal changes during menopause transition.

Menopausal transition brings significant hormonal changes, notably a decrease in estrogen, leading to vaginal dryness as a prevalent symptom. Hormonal fluctuations during breastfeeding and after childbirth can also exacerbate this condition. Additionally, certain medications, such as those for hormonal contraception or antidepressants, can further disrupt natural vaginal lubrication.

Understanding menopause as a natural phase of life is crucial. With awareness of hormonal fluctuations and bodily changes, individuals can take proactive steps to maintain comfort and confidence during this transition. Treatments like Hormone

Replacement Therapy (HRT) or procedures such as Desirial injections or Votiva Radio frequency sessions can assist in managing vaginal dryness and promoting intimate well being during this stage of life.

Embracing menopause as a natural phase enables individuals to navigate this change gracefully, supported by appropriate care and interventions. By prioritizing self-care and seeking necessary support, individuals can embrace this new chapter of life with confidence and vitality.

- **Medications**

  Some medications, such as hormonal contraceptives, antidepressants, and allergy medications, may disrupt the natural lubrication in the vaginal area. For instance, hormonal contraceptives like birth control pills, patches, or intrauterine devices (IUDs) can alter hormone levels, potentially leading to changes in vaginal moisture. Similarly, antidepressants, often prescribed for mental health conditions, can sometimes result in side effects such as vaginal dryness. It is essential to stay informed about these potential effects and discuss them with healthcare providers to consider alternative options. Additionally, certain allergy medications, particularly those containing antihistamines, might contribute to decreased lubrication. Women should be mindful of these potential side effects and their implications for intimate wellness. If you're experiencing discomfort due to your medication, it's advisable to consult your healthcare provider to explore alternative solutions.

- **Stress and Anxiety**

  Stress and anxiety can manifest in a variety of physical ways, including vaginal lubrication. Elevated levels of cortisol, known as the stress hormone, can disrupt the body's natural moisture levels, resulting in dryness and decreased responsiveness in intimate areas. Adopting effective stress management techniques can help mitigate these effects on intimate wellness. Whether through mindful practices such as: regular exercise, strong support system(s), and/ or engaging in self-care activities, finding healthy ways to reduce stress can aid in restoring balance to the body and intimate wellness. Women need to prioritize their well-being and take steps to reclaim joy and pleasure in their lives.

- **Sjögren's Syndrome**

  Sjögren's syndrome, an autoimmune disorder, primarily affecting the moisture producing glands in various parts of the body, including the vaginal glands. This condition can lead to vaginal dryness, along with dryness in the mouth and eyes. Understanding this underlying condition is crucial for effectively managing its impact on intimate health.

If you suspect you may have Sjögren's syndrome, it's imperative to seek guidance from a healthcare professional for an accurate diagnosis and to establish a comprehensive treatment plan. Collaborating closely with healthcare providers, including rheumatologists and gynecologists, ensures holistic care and support for addressing the syndrome and its effects on intimate health.

While there's no cure for Sjögren's syndrome, numerous treatment options exist to manage symptoms and alleviate vaginal dryness. Moisturizing gels or lubricants formulated explicitly for vaginal dryness can offer relief and enhance comfort during intimacy.

- **Hygiene Products**

  Attention women: when it comes to caring for our intimate areas, not all products are equally suitable. The vagina maintains a naturally acidic environment, typically with a pH level ranging between 3.8 and 4.5. However, various factors can upset this balance, resulting in dryness and irritation. Harsh soaps, douches, and scented products have the potential to disrupt the delicate pH balance, depriving the vagina of its protective moisture and leading to discomfort.

Selecting mild, pH-balanced products designed explicitly for intimate hygiene is crucial. These products aid in preserving the natural acidity of the intimate area, thereby maintaining its healthy environment. Furthermore, limiting excessive washing and choosing water-based lubricants during sexual activity can help prevent dryness and irritation. If you encounter persistent dryness or irritation, seeking advice from a healthcare professional for personalized guidance is advisable. Remember, maintaining the delicate pH balance of the vagina is essential for promoting overall vaginal health and warding off the discomfort linked with dryness and irritation.

Strategies For Managing Vaginal Dryness

Encountering vaginal dryness is a prevalent issue among women, with statistics revealing that 17% of women aged 18-50 and 34% of those over 50 experience this discomfort. However, despite its prevalence, only a mere 4% of affected women actively seek treatment, underscoring the unfortunate reality that many endure this condition silently.

The encouraging news is that solutions exist to address vaginal dryness effectively. Here are five approaches to managing this condition:

- **Hormone Replacement Therapy (HRT)**

Vaginal dryness commonly arises as a symptom of menopause due to the gradual decline in estrogen levels during the natural aging process. Hormone Replacement Therapy (HRT) emerges as a viable option in menopause management, aiming to balance hormonal levels and alleviate associated symptoms, including vaginal dryness.

- **Utilize Vaginal Treatments**

Various vaginal treatments can assist in restoring lubrication and moisture. These treatments, typically containing low-dose hormones, include:

✓ Vaginal estrogen cream

✓ Estrogen ring

✓ Tablets

- **Incorporate Vaginal Lubricants During Intimate Moments**

One of the challenges posed by vaginal dryness is its impact on intimacy. To address this, consider using lubricants during both foreplay and intercourse. Unlike topical hormone creams applied daily, these lubricants are applied before intercourse. It's crucial to choose products explicitly formulated for lubrication during intercourse. Note: that while water based lubricants don't compromise condom integrity, oil-based ones increase the risk of condom tears, sheet stains, and infections.

- **Body Care Products**

Surprisingly, body care products can exacerbate vaginal dryness by irritating vaginal tissues. Fragrances and harsh cleansing agents found in soap, body wash, and laundry detergent may contain ingredients contributing to dryness. Avoid using vaginal washes and douche, as they can lead to irritation, dryness, and potential infections by disrupting beneficial flora.

The U.S. Department of Health & Human Services recommends the following for vaginal hygiene:

- Wash the exterior of the vagina with warm water (mild soap may contribute to dryness).
- Avoid scented products, including pads and tampons.

Remember, the vagina is self-cleaning, and excessive cleansing can disrupt its natural balance. As estrogen levels decline during menopause, so too does vaginal moisture, leaving many women feeling like they're stuck in the desert without a canteen. Fear not, dear readers, for we've got some tricks up our sleeves to help you reclaim your comfort and confidence in the bedroom. From lubricants to moisturizers, there's a whole arsenal of products designed to keep things slippery when wet - because, let's face it, nobody likes feeling like they're trying to navigate the Sahara during sex.

It's not just about physical discomfort - menopause can also impact your libido and desire for intimacy. As your hormones go haywire, so too can our sexual appetite, leaving many women feeling like they've lost that loving feeling. Please don't fret, my fellow menopausal mavens, for there are plenty of ways to reignite the spark in the bedroom. Feel free to try everything from exploring new forms of intimacy to communicating openly with your partner about your needs and desires, there's no shortage of ways to keep the flames of passion burning bright - even amid menopause.

Keep in mind that there's still plenty of fun to be had in the bedroom, even if it feels like your hormones are playing a cruel joke on you. So grab your fans because we're about to dive into the wild world of menopausal intimacy with ten tips to keep the flames of passion burning bright:

- **Lubrication, Lubrication:** Think of lubricant as your new best friend – the kind that never judges you for needing a little extra help in the moisture department. Keep a bottle handy (or ten), and don't be afraid to apply liberally. Slippery when wet has never been more relevant!

- **Foreplay, Foreplay, Foreplay:** Menopause may have thrown your hormones for a loop, but that doesn't mean you can't still enjoy the journey. Take your time with plenty of foreplay to get the engines revving and set the mood for a night of passion.

- **Communicate Like a Pro:** Your partner isn't a mind reader (unless they've suddenly developed telepathic powers, in which case, please share your secret), so don't be afraid to communicate openly about your needs, desires, and any discomfort you may be experiencing.

- **Get Creative:** Menopause may have damaged things, but it's also an opportunity to get creative in the bedroom. Explore new positions, toys, and fantasies to keep things fresh and exciting.

- **Set the Mood:** Dim the lights, light some candles, and put on your favorite sexy playlist – creating the right ambiance can make all the difference in setting the stage for a night of passion.

- **Take Care of Yourself:** Self-care isn't just about face masks and bubble baths – it's also about taking care of your sexual health. Eat well, exercise regularly, and prioritize sleep to keep your hormones in check and your libido humming.

- **Laugh It Off:** Sometimes, you have to laugh at the absurdity of it all. Embrace the quirks of menopause with humor, and remember that laughter truly is the best medicine - especially when navigating intimacy's ups and downs.

- **Explore New Avenues of Pleasure:** Menopause may have closed one door, but it's opened plenty of others. Take this opportunity to explore new avenues of pleasure - whether it's through solo play, mutual masturbation, or trying out new kinks with your partner.

- **Stay Positive:** Menopause can be challenging, but it's also a chance to embrace your body and all its quirks. Stay positive, focus on the things you love about yourself, and remember that you're still a sexual goddess - hot flashes and all.

- **Seek Professional Help If Needed:** If you're experiencing persistent discomfort or issues with intimacy, don't hesitate to seek help from a healthcare professional. There are plenty of treatments and therapies available to help you reclaim your sexual health and enjoyment - so don't suffer in silence!

So there you have it: Pro tips for enjoying intimacy during menopause. Remember, you're not alone in this journey. With a bit of humor, creativity, and a lot of lubricant, you can keep the fires of passion burning bright – even amid the hormonal rollercoaster of menopause.

———————— ♂ ————————

As we bid farewell to this whirlwind exploration of intimacy during menopause, let's take a moment to reflect on the journey we've embarked upon together--from navigating the hormonal rollercoaster to embracing new forms of pleasure, we've laughed, learned, and perhaps even blushed a time or two along the way.

Yet, amidst the hot flashes and mood swings, one thing remains abundantly clear: menopause may bring its fair share of challenges, but it also presents an opportunity for growth, exploration, and, yes, even a little bit of fun in the bedroom. So, as you enter the world armed with lubricant, laughter, and a newfound sense of confidence, remember that you are not alone in this journey.

Whether flying solo or exploring with a partner, may you embrace the ups and downs of menopausal intimacy with grace, humor, and a healthy dose of self-love. After all, life is too short to let a little thing like menopause get in the way of pleasure, passion, and the pursuit of happiness.

So here's to you, dear reader – may your journey through menopause be filled with laughter, love, and plenty of mind-blowing moments in the bedroom. After all, if there's one thing menopause has taught us, there's always room for a little more excitement in our lives – especially when it comes to matters of the heart (and other body parts).

Common Vaginal Concerns: From A To Z

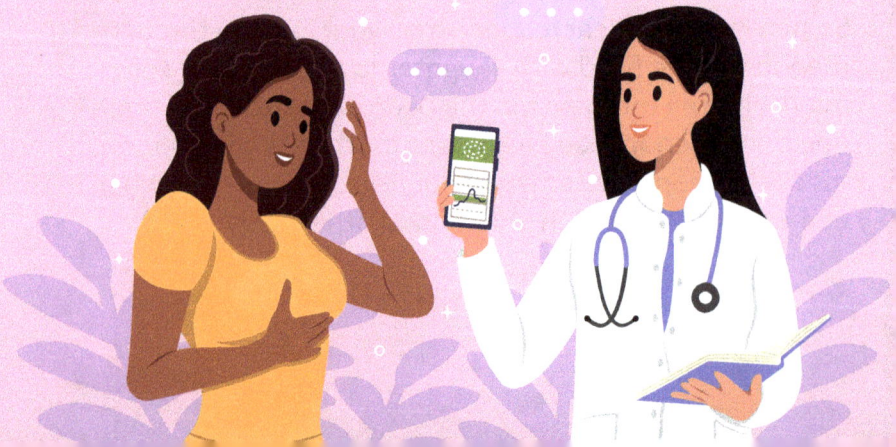

Common Vaginal Concerns is such an intriguing subject that can be a little awkward to talk about, but that should not worry you, as we are going on to this adventurous and fantastic journey into the world of common vaginal concerns.

Just imagine: It's another day and you're just doing your thing when all of a sudden, you feel itchy in one spot or another or worse, maybe it's some burning sensation, some strange smells or even that discomforting feeling that simply refuses to let go. However it happens, it's obvious that there is something on your lady parts which wants to communicate with you; thus listen up.

In this chapter, we will explore various issues affecting women down there with commonest being yeast infections as well as unwanted intruders like jock itch and crabs. You should however not worry because by the time you are done with this chapter, having gained knowledge out of it and being lighthearted about it all, you will be ready for any vaginal challenge.

Therefore, be prepared for a new experience in understanding vaginal health better than ever before. This means knowing how to handle stubborn yeast infections and UTIs as well as eliminating jock itch and crabs from your private parts among other areas. When it is finally inevitable that you have to swallow hard for once then arrange an embarrassing appointment with your gynecologist, rest assured in the fact that we shall accompany you all the way through this process.

Indeed no health matter or even one regarding one's personal wellbeing is considered off limits particularly where lady bits are involved!

──────── ♂ ────────

Vaginal Ailments

Your body is like a sacred temple, whereas vaginal problems are like uninvited guests who crash parties in this private house of yours. These disease conditions may cause severe life disruptions, make you uncomfortable and even embarrass you. Do not be afraid with knowledge and a pinch of humor, you can maneuver the vagaries of vaginal health.

Unfortunately, there are several vaginal issues from the annoying itchiness of yeast infections (vulvovaginal candidiasis) to the painful burning sensation that accompanies urinary tract infections (UTIs) that can leave one feeling less than ideal. Even so, understanding what's going on down there is the first step toward finding relief and reclaiming your comfort. Remember we've got you covered every step of the way, from recognizing the symptoms to exploring the best ways to treat and prevent these pesky ailments.

- **Vaginal Candidiasis (Yeast Infection)**

You're having your day as usual when suddenly an itch hits you out of nowhere. It might be accompanied by a thick white discharge that looks like cottage cheese. Yay! You have just been initiated into a yeast infection caused by Candida fungus overgrowth.

The primary cause for yeast infection is an overgrowth of Candida albicans which is a type of fungi naturally found in the vagina. This situation may be caused by several factors such as hormonal changes (e.g., pregnancy, menstruation), antibiotic use, weakened immune system, diabetes, or tight clothing.

The symptoms include: itching, a burning sensation, redness and swelling in the vulva area, curdy white thick discharge from the vagina similar to cottage cheese and discomfort during sexual intercourse or while urinating. Normally treatment involves antifungal medication in form of creams / ointments / suppositories / oral tablets. Over-the-counter antifungal medications which are available but if they do not work well for stubborn/ severe infections doctors prescribe stronger ones. For example, patients must finish their whole course of treatment even if there's an improvement in symptoms so that a relapse doesn't occur.

- **Urinary Tract Infections (UTIs)**

This is a common problem for most women. UTIs may develop when bacteria, commonly Escherichia coli (E. coli) from the digestive tract, enter and breed in the urinary system causing infection. Factors that increase the likelihood of contracting a UTI include: sexual activity, improper cleansing after defecation especially by wiping the anus from behind towards front, holding urine for too long, using catheters to pass urine, going through menopause and specific illnesses like diabetes.

The signs of a UTI can be: a strong, urgent need to urinate constantly, burning feeling during urination; passing small amounts of urine on frequent basis; cloudy or bloody urine; foul smell after urination; pelvic pain and occasional fever or chills.

Treatment for UTIs involves administration of antibiotics. Selection choice and duration of antibiotic therapy depends on factors such as: severity of symptoms, type of bacteria responsible for infection and medical history of patient. These solutions can help decrease signs as well as prevent future occurrences: consuming large amounts water, frequently emptying bladder and limiting substances capable upsetting it e.g., alcohol coffee spices among others. Further examination and strategies to prevent is recommended in cases of recurring urinary tract infections.

- **Bacterial Vaginosis**

You may not know that bacterial vaginosis (BV) is more widespread than you might think.

Bacterial vaginosis arises when there is an imbalance between harmful bacteria in the vagina and normal vaginal flora bacteria. Although the reason behind BV isn't always known, some things like douching, multiple sexual partners, new sexual partners, and certain hygiene products may cause disruption in vaginal PH leading to BV.

It is possible for many women with BV to have no symptoms at all. However those who notice anything abnormal about their genital regions tend to have white or grayish thin fluids which mostly have a fishy smell after sex. Some women may also experience itching or irritation around the vagina. In most cases, BV is treated with antibiotics such as metronidazole or clindamycin. These drugs can be taken by mouth, inserted into the vagina or given in gel form. Simultaneous treatment of sexual partners is important to prevent re-infection. Stop douching and using scented hygiene products to avoid recurrence.

- **Trichomoniasis**

This crafty parasite is sometimes discreet but can be extremely obvious. Trichomoniasis is a sexually transmitted illness that develops when a woman gets infected with Trichomonas vaginalis, a parasite. It spreads through sexual intercourse with an individual who already has it. Multiple sex partners, unprotected sex and history of STIs are among factors that increase the risk of trichomoniasis.

Symptoms may differ, but usually include frothy yellow-green discharge from the vagina which smells bad. In women, this could lead to itching in the vagina as well as irritation. They may also feel pain during urination or while having sex which can cause redness down there or discomfort during sexual intercourse. Others may have lower abdominal pain or spotting between periods.

Antibiotics like metronidazole and tinidazole are used to treat trichomoniasis by killing off the parasites in the blood stream. Sexually active people should both be treated at the same time to avoid re-infection. Once treatment is completed and symptoms cease patients should abstain from any sexual contact until treatment completion so that they do not pass on these germs.

- **Atrophy (Atrophic Vaginitis)**

Reduced levels of estrogen primarily because of menopause or due to medical procedures such as radiation therapy and chemotherapy can cause vaginal dryness and atrophy most commonly occurs. The hormone estrogen keeps vaginal walls thick and strong and helps produce natural lubrication for the vagina. When estrogen decreases, thinning of vaginal tissues due to drying out happens while they become less elastic making them susceptible to irritations and inflammations.

Some common symptoms are: vaginitis including dryness, itching, burning sensations; dyspareunia including some pain or discomfort during intercourse; postcoital bleeding; vaginitis such as soreness or irritation; high chances of urinary tract infections.

———————— ♂ ————————

Therapy for vaginal dryness/atrophic vaginitis places emphasis on adding moisture into the vagina and restoring healthy tissues. For example, there are over-the-counter vaginal moisturizers or lubricants. Other forms of treatment include topical estrogen in form of tablets, creams or rings; or systemic estrogen therapy for menopausal women. Regular sexual intercourse or using dilators could be advised to maintain vaginal elasticity and reduce pain during sexual activity. In determining the most appropriate treatment for a patient, healthcare professionals will need to take into account the individuals medical history as well as any specific needs they may have.

Prevention is Key: However most of these common vaginal afflictions may seem like an annoyance, there is something that can be done to stop them before they start occurring. This may mean avoiding irritating substances such as scented soap and douches, good hygienic practices and changes in daily routine. When unsure about anything related to your vagina's health, contact a healthcare professional who will give directions because it's their area of expertise.

The Itch That Won't Quit

Jock itch is the first thing I want to discuss. Imagine that you have just finished a long workout at your favorite gym and feel like a champion when you are suddenly greeted with an itching feeling in your genital area. Yes, this is jock itch. A fungal infection that thrives in warm and damp places. To get rid of this nuisance one must do more than throw away the gym shorts alone. We will be talking about what jock itch is, how it is transmitted (hint: athletes are not the only ones) and most importantly how one can get rid of it. Some of the remedies include: antifungal creams to keeping roomy undies around your 'danglies', we've got all the tips and tricks you need to kick moisture out of here.

To fully comprehend jock itch, you have to know what it entails. Tinea cruris as it is known scientifically is an annoying fungal infection which resides on moist areas such as the groin leading to its ideal breeding ground. Anyone can end up being affected by this condition whether they are regular users of gym or people who sweat excessively or any sports freaks among us. However, there are ways one can keep these uninvited guests away.

Have no fear for you can actually banish jock itch from under your belly button down below where the sun doesn't shine. Firstly, ensure you always keep the area clean and dry. After bathing or sweating make sure you dry yourself off completely before wearing fresh cotton underwear. This process will allow for circulation of air since most sweat pants retain moisture inside them, thus causing itching, odor and irritation which can be caused by chaffing. Second, as far as over-the-counter medications go, antifungal creams are best for getting rid of this infection; these creams work towards killing the fungus causing jock itch thereby giving relief from itching and reducing inflammation.

Now let's move on to pubic lice- those tiny creatures that could cause big problems in your nether regions. Pubic lice are tiny insects that feed on human blood and are also known as crab lice. They are transmitted through intimate contact such as sexual relations or by sharing towels or bed clothes; they can quickly infest the pubic hair causing severe itching and discomfort.

For effective treatment, it is important to know the signs of pubic lice. You should be able to notice small insects shaped like crabs in public hairs and even tiny white eggs called nits attached to the hair shafts. Moreover, another symptom of an infestation with pubic lice is an itchiness in the genital area. With that being said, if you believe that you may have contracted pubic lice don't start looking for a desert island to live on – there are many treatments that can help. Over-the-counter treatments like medicated shampoos and lotions offer some relief from this condition by eliminating the parasites including their eggs too. Just ensure you follow all instructions carefully while washing your linen or clothing which could be affected.

However, despite jock itch and pubic lice being unwelcome guests below the belt, they can be defeated. Once armed with awareness and proper hygienic practices plus appropriate therapy one can frustrate these critters out their discomfort zone. So, don't let jock itch or pubic lice get best of you but instead confront them head-on, showing whose boss!

Swallow Your Pride

Let's start by looking into this uncomfortable yet important aspect of keeping our vagina healthy. It is known that booking an appointment with your gynecologist can be a source of embarrassment, anxiety or shame for many women. The idea of sharing intimate details about one's body with a total stranger can be daunting to put it mildly. Nonetheless, in the name of your health especially vaginal health, these feelings must be overcome and we should look out for ourselves.

Firstly, it is important to realize that you are not alone in feeling anxious about visiting a gynecologist. Many females experience similar uneasiness or awkwardness; this is normal. Our society has often shied away from discussing issues relating to reproductive health, making them taboo subjects such as menstruation, sexual activity and others. On the other hand, when acknowledged and accepted, it's possible to overcome them and embark on proactive measures towards caring for one's body.

The biggest obstacle for women while seeking medical help in respect to vaginal health is fear of condemnation or humiliation. Whether afraid of being criticized for their sexual history, hygiene practices or symptoms exhibited by one's body; these concerns do make it difficult for one to ask for assistance. Nevertheless, one must always remember that gynecologists are medical professionals who have committed their lives to assisting women concerning their reproductive health matters. They have seen and heard it all and are trained to provide compassionate care which lacks judgementalism unlike what some patients think.

Further, another common reason why women shy away from going for gyno visits is fear of bad news or negative diagnosis. Sure, there may be some apprehension about getting scary results during an examination but it should be noted that early detection plays a key role in dealing with any possible ailments before they get out of hand. Ignoring the symptoms or even avoiding the doctor only exacerbates the problem further leading to more serious conditions later on in life. One must take charge of their health and enabling oneself to make informed decisions about one's care is vital.

In the end, making that appointment with a gynecologist despite feeling ashamed or afraid is an act of self-love and self-advocacy. It's all about putting one's health and well being first even if it doesn't feel comfortable or safe. By making sure that you schedule regular check-ups to address any concerns, you are being proactive in maintaining peak vaginal health as well as general well-being. So take a deep breath, pick up the phone, and remember that you're doing something good for yourself and future self will thank you for it!

The Importance Of Regular Checkups

A visit to your gynecologist is not just a routine; it is one of the most important steps in proactive care for women. These visits act as preventative measures that enable healthcare providers to monitor your vaginal health and identify any possible problems early. To understand more deeply why these exams are so vital. Let's discuss below:

- **Early identification of issues**
  Regular check-ups allow gynecologists to perform thorough examinations such as pelvic exams and pap smears, which can detect abnormalities or signs of infections. Early detection increases the chances of successful treatment and reduces complications. Most cases of cervical cancer,

sexually transmitted diseases (STDs) and pelvic inflammatory disease (PID), for instance, are usually asymptomatic in their initial stages but can be detected through regular screenings for early intervention and control.

- **Individualized Care and Support**

  By going for regular checkups, a woman's OB-GYN provides her with personalized care that suits her specific concerns and needs. Regardless if a woman has menstrual irregularities, needs birth control methods or menopause guidance, the medical professional will guide her accordingly. Any such consultations offer an excellent chance to talk about anything concerning reproduction health that might be troubling her. An OB-GYN may provide scientific based information as well as help dispel myths and provide recommendations to enhance her wellbeing.

- **Whole Health Assessment**

  Routine genital checks encompass more than just vaginal health because they take into account the general appraisal of one's overall wellness and physical conditions. This involves finding out about the person's personal history, lifestyle factors or any changes since last time they visited a specialist in this field. By doing this comprehensive examination healthcare providers can spot potential risk factors before they begin developing into something severe. Thus when such clinical meetings occur discussions on sexual health promotion may be conducted alongside mental health topic including preventive measures like immunizations so that all facets of ones' wellbeing receive satisfactory attention.

- **Empowerment via Knowledge**

  Beyond diagnosis and treatment, regular checkups empower women through education and awareness. Reproductive anatomy, menstruation, contraception, prevention of STIs and others are some of the things women can learn from their gynecologists. Knowing one's body and what it requires helps one to make informed choices concerning one's health. It is also possible to have conversations on how to change one's way of life in relation to dieting, exercising and managing stress, subsequently, ensuring health and youthfulness.

- **Building Trust**

  Developing a bond with one's OB-GYN through regular checkups creates an atmosphere of trust and respect for both parties involved. This relationship is important when it comes to free expression as well as talking about sensitive topics without feeling judged or being ashamed. With time, the professional becomes familiar with one's medical history alongside their likes and dislikes coupled with other unique matters related to them which in turn helps the OB-GYN personalize their care.

To sum up, regular check-ups with a gynecologist are foundational for women who stand to gain more than just vaginal care services from such visits. In so doing they take proactive steps towards protecting their reproductive system, identifying problems early on, and receiving specialized counsel from doctors. Please do not underrate the significance of going for routine checks –your path towards a healthy life is based on them. So don't neglect regular check-ups; they are your doorway to well-being at its best.

9

Self-Care For Down There

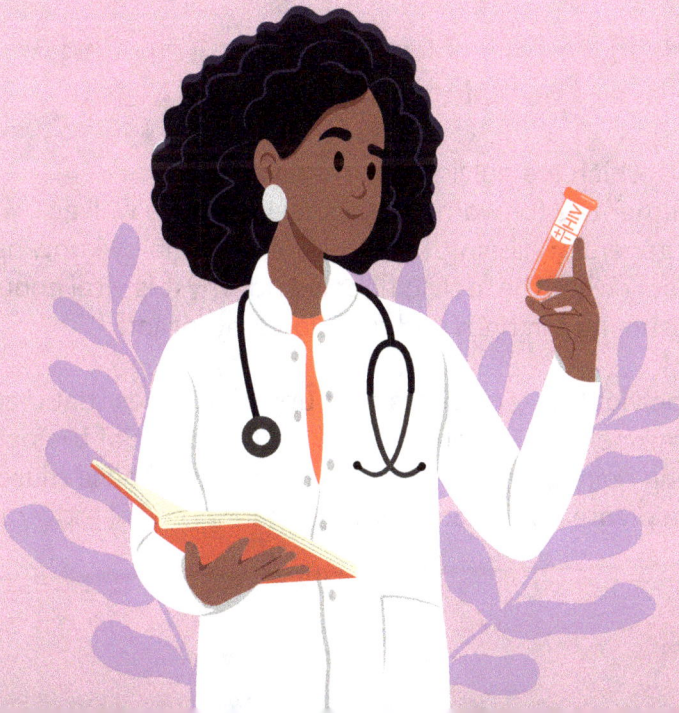

*A*ll right, let's talk about the elephant in the room or should I say, the 'pussy' in the room? In terms of self-care, we often concentrate on our skin, hair and mental health but what about 'down there'? Yes, your vagina- that powerhouse of femininity that is usually a shadow position in our self-care routines. Howbeit, if revealed to you that attending to your lady parts is equally essential- if not more than those weekly face masks or sessions of yoga?

Be ready to question established norms and start an enlightenment path accompanied by some breaking of taboos with it, because our vaginas also deserve care folks. Some of which involves--becoming a Kegel queen due to pelvic floor exercises, to how stress affects your lady bits- we are now going into the world of vaginal self-care. So grab a hot cup of tea while you get cozy and prepare yourself for giving tender loving care to "down there".

Pelvic Floor Exercises And Other Self-Care Practices For Maintaining Vaginal Health.

Kegels which are pelvic floor exercises serve as fundamentals for women's vaginal health as well as their general wellbeing. However, let us begin by knowing precisely what the pelvic floor is and why it is vital enough to ensure its strength and function stay intact.

The pelvic floor represents a groups of muscles that create a hammock-like structure at the bottom part of the pelvis helping hold up bladder, uterus and rectum. These muscles play a pivotal role in controlling urination, bowel movement and sexual function too. Nevertheless, factors such as childbirth, aging, obesity and chronic strain could weaken these muscles leading to various problems such urinary incontinence (UI), prolapsed pelvic organ disease (POP) coupled with diminished sexual satisfaction.

This brings us to pelvic floor exercise known as Kegels. Invented by doctor Arnold Kegel during 1940s it entails contracting and releasing these muscle groups for the purpose of enhancing their strength, sustainability and coordination. Continuously practicing this exercise can help avert or reduce incidences of urinary incontinence, hold up pelvic organs, and heighten sexual pleasure as well as aid in post-birth recovery.

Therefore, how do you do Kegels? It's elementary! Firstly, identify your target muscles which are the ones that would make you stop urinating mid-flow or hold it when you feel like farting. Once determined, contract these muscles as if you were trying to lift them upwards and inwards. Hold this contraction for a few seconds before relaxing and releasing it. Aim at doing them ten to fifteen times daily taking three cycles.

However, there is more to pelvic floor health than just Kegels. There are other self-care practices that boost what this exercise can achieve. For example, keeping off pounds helps to relieve pressure on your pelvic floor while avoiding constipation prevents straining too much during defecation that causes weakening of muscles over time.

—————— ♂ ——————

The role of a balanced diet in overall health, including vaginal health should not be underestimated. A complete diet comprising fruits, vegetables, whole grains and lean meats, is full of nutrients and antioxidants that enable immune function and maintain a healthy environment for the vagina. Foods such as yogurt, kefir and sauerkraut are rich in probiotics which help to keep the natural bacteria balance in check thereby reducing the chances of infections such as bacterial vaginosis or yeast infection. Besides, water is an essential element of life because it helps to eliminate toxins from our bodies; this applies even to the body's genitals.

Moreover, maintaining good posture and body mechanics can also protect your pelvic floor from unnecessary strain and harm. Therefore, whenever you lift something heavy, it is important to bend with knees straight while keeping back upright so that you do not put pressure on the pelvic muscles unnecessarily.

Maintaining proper hygiene is very important when it comes to preventing infections as well as keeping the vagina healthy. But remember; there has to be a balance since too much washing or using harsh soaps can disrupt the natural pH levels in your vagina causing irritation and infections. Instead go for mild cleansers without fragrance made specifically for use in private parts and avoid douching; this will help prevent flushing out beneficial bacteria and minimize chances of getting infected. The genital area outside should be washed everyday with warm water plus mild soap while wiping from front towards back after using toilet facilities can limit transmission of harmful bacteria from anus towards vagina.

───────── ♂ ─────────

To protect vaginal and overall health, practicing safe sex is crucial. Sex can cause sexually transmitted infections (STIs) and other complications when not protected. Key safe sex practices include:

Condom Use: Consistently employ condoms during vaginal, oral and anal sex for a decrease in the possibility of STIs such as HIV, gonorrhea, chlamydia and genital herpes.

Regular STI Testing: Frequent testing for STIs is necessary especially if one has multiple sexual partners or involves in risky sexual behavior. Detecting and treating STIs in good time helps avoid future problems and protects personal well-being.

Communication: Talk openly with your sexual partners about your history of STI's and test regularly to prevent these diseases from being passed on to others. Healthy sexual relationships are based on mutual respect and trust thus reducing chances of contracting STI's.

Moreover, relaxation techniques that involve deep breathing exercises, yoga or mindful meditation can be adopted as part of routine activities to reduce stress levels within the pelvic region hence improving muscle function with the general wellbeing of the vagina.

Therefore, pelvic floor exercises coupled with other types of self-care practices are very important ways through which women may maintain their vaginal health while preventing disorders related to pelvic floor. You'll feel more confident every day by being proactive about strengthening your pelvic floor muscles.

Effects Of Stress On Your Lady Parts And Why You Need To Prioritize Relaxation & Self-Care

Stress not only takes a toll on our mental state but also affects our overall physical well being including our vaginal health. Our bodies release stress hormones like cortisol and adrenaline when we get stressed out which can disrupt this delicate balance.

A silent saboteur of our well-being – Stress is commonly associated with headaches, insomnia or even digestive issues but we rarely pay attention how it affects our lady parts/organs. Make no mistake about it; just like any other organ in the body stress will have some impacts on vaginal health.

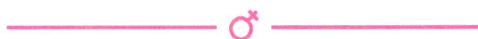

———————— ♂ ————————

In the first place, let us examine how stress affects the body in a physiological level. When we're stressed out, our bodies go into overdrive and flood our system with stress hormones such as cortisol and adrenaline. These hormones, though good for short term use, can have serious side effects when they are left to course through our veins unchecked.

The most visible impact of chronic stress on lady parts is an imbalance of hormones in the body. On one hand, elevated levels of stress hormones like cortisol can disrupt the balance between estrogen and progesterone causing irregular menstrual cycles, alterations in vaginal discharge or even impinging on sex drive.

Furthermore, it can also lower immunity that makes women more susceptible to infections such as yeast infections or bacterial vaginosis (BV). Opportunistic pathogens take advantage of weakened immune defenses that otherwise regulate a delicate balance between bacteria and yeast within the vagina leading to several complications.

However, it's not only physical factors of stress that affect our lady parts; there is also a psychological side to it. Stress leads to anxiety disorders, depression and low self-esteem which all negatively affect sexual health among individuals. In situations where one is constantly under high amounts of anxiety or pressure then there are natural tendencies towards becoming distant with their own bodies as well as shying away from intimacy which just adds on issues such as vaginal dryness during sex leading further discomfort.

Well, what is it? It is simple - prioritize relaxation and self-care. A vaginal health necessity, rather than a luxury, unwinding and distressing your mind from the day's activities can help you with this. Be it mindful meditation, yoga, deep breathing exercises or simply doing things that make you happy; finding ways to deal with stress should be an important aspect of keeping a healthy balance in your lady parts.

Your vagina deserves just as much care and attention as the rest of your body. By making relaxation and self-care a priority, you are not only improving your vaginal health but also investing in your overall well-being and happiness.

Body Positivity And Learning To Love The Skin You're In

Living in a world full of unrealistic beauty standards and airbrushing, appreciating ones– body quirks, curves and all– can be seen as an act of self-love that is rebellious. However, when it comes to our female genitalia this may involve a more intricate journey challenging societal taboos that requires us to possess our own bodies again.

First things first: Your body is an incredible work of art; a masterpiece formed by the intricate play of genetics, environment, and personal history. All this from the curve of your hips to the gentle folds of your labia, each part plays its own special role towards overall health and vitality.

Nevertheless, many women grow up feeling detached from their bodies because they are taught to see themselves from a perspective created by shame or not being enough. We are repeatedly exposed to messages that communicate unacceptability in relation to our bodies; too fat, too thin, too hairy or wrinkled leaving an endless battle with one's own reflection.

Your most loyal companion on life's journey is not your enemy but your body itself. Therefore, when it comes embracing what you have between legs you should appreciate the uniqueness exhibited by them and their capability for joy and pleasure even after facing hardships in their lives.

To embark upon this path towards self-acceptance and body positivity though we need to take certain steps. First of all try changing how you see things —particularly negative talk about ourselves that constantly occurs within your minds. Instead fixate on what you can do with it—its pleasurable experiences, its procreative ability as well as strength rather than perceived shortcomings or defects.

As such surround yourself with positive influences such as body-positive role models, supportive friends, empowering social media accounts (which make sure they celebrate diversity) until you're passing like this...you only live once: I guess Living La Vida Loca would be highly appropriate at this point. Remember that other people are also going through the same thing as you and that makes us strong when we come together.

Lastly, practice extreme self-love by treating yourself with kindness, compassion, and respect. Whether it means having a luxurious bubble bath, eating your favorite dessert guilt-free or just looking at yourself in the mirror while saying "I love you," self-care must be part of your daily routine.

Thus, embracing your body is not solely about accepting it physically but rather realizing its intrinsic worth, strength, resilience and capability for change. By lovingly accepting your lady parts, you aren't just claiming ownership over your body but also reclaiming your power and embracing all things beautiful about yourself.

10

Putting It All Together: Your Vagina, Your Rules

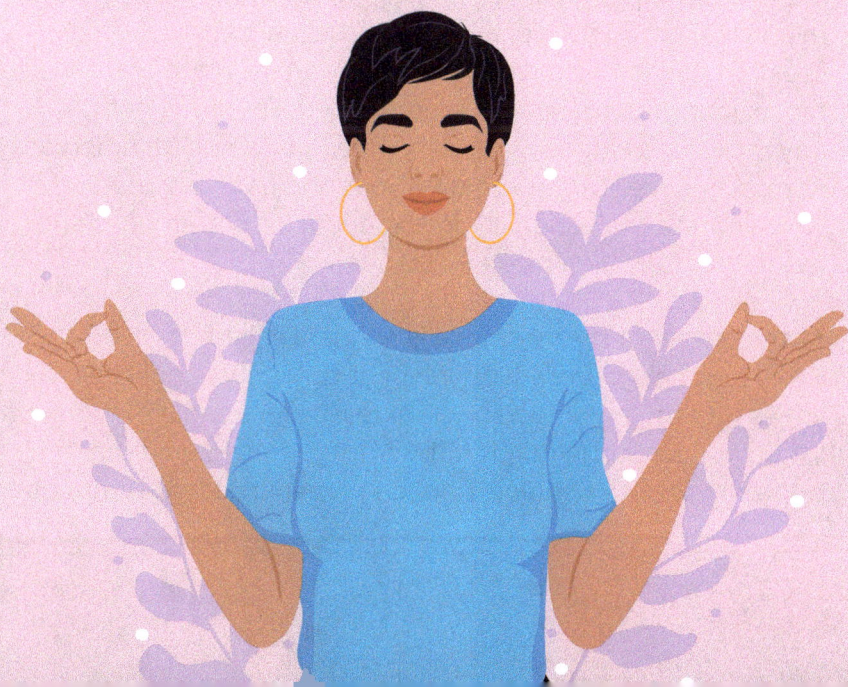

Your private part, your own principles. Although brief, this phrase means a lot to anyone who is struggling with complex issues of feminine health. This world is full of suggestions and societal demands making it difficult for one to even know what is good for her body. Nevertheless, in the chaos of noises there is one truth that stands firm; every individual has absolute authority over their vaginal well-being.

We have explored female anatomy, debunked myths surrounding it and looked at various vaginal problems that exist from puberty to menopause, from hygiene to intimacy. We are now here in the final chapter where we have approached a major milestone - reminding ourselves on how our vaginas should never be judged or controlled by outsiders other than being vessels of self-expression, resilience and autonomy.

The point of this section is simple yet very significant: you are the captain of your vagina ship. Choosing the right menstrual products, defending your sexual satisfaction or seeking medical help when necessary are all up to you as far as your vagina's health is concerned. There will not be any more restrictions by society on what can be regarded as normal or acceptable regarding your bodies today. Instead, we celebrate the variability in experiences, preferences and requirements which make us unique.

At the center of this message is an ideal called "choice." Every person's journey with respect to their vaginal health varies depending on personal values, beliefs and situations. What works for one might not work for another and that's perfectly fine! The choice between organic cotton tampons and reusable menstrual cups isn't important; neither does shaving off public hair matter compared to leaving it bushy - both choices do matter!

However, having choices alone cannot bring about change. In a world still filled with misinformation and stigma around conversations about vaginal health; open communication has become imperative. We must create spaces where conversations flow freely without limitations or barriers only allowing relevant questions to arise within them. Together we enable each other through sharing stories of our struggles, successes and failures thereby creating opportunities for collective growth and understanding.

Supportive communities are also important as illustrated in this chapter. These are groups of like-minded persons serving as sounding boards who share experiences with us. They could either be online or offline, but their purpose is to offer guidance, information and celebrate our bodies without shame or fear. We join hands shouting in unison for a change towards the status quo where every person's vagina health is appreciated.

As we take on this last part of our journey, let us raise our glasses to acknowledge the inherent strength and extraordinary resilience in each one of us. Cheers to loving our vaginas wholeheartedly with compassion and unwavering certainty. Cheers to breaking ground on your terms, drawing lines for yourself and living with the maxim: "Your vagina, your rules."

Our Vagina, Your Choice

One principle is preeminent among others in matters of vaginal health: autonomy. You alone own your vagina, and you control it. This goes beyond the anatomical perspective; it includes choices, limits, and priorities that drive your experience with vaginal health.

The most crucial concept to consider in terms of vaginal health is autonomy; this gives individuals power to own their bodies, make informed decisions and assert their rights. Autonomy means realizing that no one has the right to dictate or invalidate your choices regarding what happens to your vagina.

Drawing boundaries and setting priorities are fundamental tenets of self-care and empowerment within the realm of vaginal health. This means understanding what matters to you, which can include values, needs, or limits that require immediate action towards protection and prioritization of you as an individual. Here's why setting boundaries and priorities in vaginal health matters:

1. Protection From Harm

Boundaries act as a protective shield around yourself and your vaginal wellness; they spell out what is acceptable or not in various contexts such as intimate relationships, medical encounters or self-care practices for example.

2. Self-Rule Continuation

Your ability to preserve your autonomy as well as agency over your body mainly depends on having certain boundaries in place. In other words, whether it involves refusing some medical treatments, limiting sexual activities or asserting yourself medically when seeking help, it's all about drawing lines that respects oneself.

3. Well-Being Enhancement

You may have reasons for putting all efforts into maintaining good health related to your vagina. To begin with this might include: aspects like satisfaction, protection against infections, fertility, etc. Also, by making major concerns among them; we are able to channel our time, energy, and resources towards overall well-being. Thus frequent bathing and exercise may be remedies for vaginal infections and then sexual pleasure and love making be given importance as well.

4. Self-Assertion And Advocacy

Setting boundaries and priorities within the context of vaginal health is an expression of your empowerment and self-defense. This calls for self-awareness, assertiveness, and bravery in demanding that your needs are met with dignity and respect. By advocating for yourself, you challenge societal norms, dispel myths, and break down barriers to accessing quality care and support. In this way, you not only stand out as a role model in terms of individual well-being but also create space for others to do the same.

5. Self-Cultivation

It is essential to promote resilience while taking oneself into account and establishing boundaries and intentions. It helps develop a framework through which stress can be managed; challenges can be tackled more successfully; while mental and psychological safety are maintained. One only gains self-esteem by knowing their boundaries, thereby creating their own worthiness resulting in overall personal development. So when it involves activities that are draining, when no time is invested into one's own relaxation, or rather if one gets assistance when necessary, prioritizing which limits come first, builds resilience, consequently creating a wholesome life.

Finding Your Tribe

The first step in finding your tribe is breaking the silence surrounding vaginal health and engaging in open, honest conversations about topics that have long been considered taboo. By normalizing discussions about menstruation, sexual pleasure, vaginal hygiene, and reproductive health, we create space for individuals to share their experiences without fear of judgment or stigma.

Open communication fosters a sense of community, allowing individuals to exchange insights, seek advice, and offer support to one another. Whether it's discussing the latest menstrual products, sharing tips for managing vaginal discomfort, or debunking myths about sexual health, these conversations help to demystify vaginal health and empower individuals to take control of their own well-being.

Moreover, open communication promotes education and awareness, enabling individuals to make informed decisions about their bodies and health care. By sharing accurate information and dispelling misconceptions, we empower ourselves and others to seek the care and support they need, leading to better outcomes and improved quality of life.

Supportive communities play a vital role in promoting holistic vaginal health and well being. Whether online or in-person, these communities offer a safe space for individuals to connect, share their stories, and seek guidance from others who understand their experiences firsthand.

One of the key benefits of supportive communities is the sense of belonging and validation they provide. Knowing that you're not alone in your experiences can be incredibly comforting and empowering, especially when facing challenges or uncertainties related to vaginal health. By connecting with others who share similar concerns and experiences, individuals can find solace, solidarity, and strength in numbers.

Supportive communities also offer practical benefits, such as access to valuable resources, expert advice, and peer support networks. Whether it's recommending a trusted gynecologist, sharing information about effective treatments, or providing emotional support during difficult times, these communities can be invaluable sources of guidance and assistance.

Furthermore, supportive communities foster a culture of empowerment and advocacy, encouraging individuals to take an active role in their own health care and become champions for change within their communities. By amplifying their voices, sharing their stories, and advocating for improved access to care and resources, community members can drive meaningful progress and create positive change in the realm of vaginal health.

Tips For Connecting With Like-Minded Individuals And Resources

So, how can you find your tribe and connect with like-minded individuals and resources? Here are some practical tips to help you get started:

Join online communities and forums dedicated to vaginal health and wellness. Platforms such as social media groups, online forums, and community websites provide opportunities to connect with others, share experiences, and access valuable resources and information.

Attend local support groups, workshops, or events focused on women's health and wellness. These gatherings offer opportunities to meet others face-to-face, engage in meaningful discussions, and form lasting connections with individuals who share your interests and concerns.

Reach out to trusted friends, family members, or healthcare providers for recommendations and referrals to supportive communities and resources. Personal referrals can be a valuable way to discover new resources and connect with individuals who understand your unique needs and experiences.

Consider seeking professional guidance from therapists, counselors, or support groups specializing in women's health and wellness. These professionals can provide personalized support, guidance, and resources to help you navigate your vaginal health journey with confidence and clarity.

Be proactive in fostering connections and building relationships within your community. Whether it's attending events, volunteering, or joining local organizations, actively engaging with others can help you expand your social network and discover new opportunities for support and collaboration.

By taking these proactive steps and embracing the power of community, you can find your tribe, cultivate meaningful connections, and embark on a journey of empowerment, education, and self-discovery in the realm of vaginal health. Together, we can create a world where every individual feels supported, informed, and empowered to prioritize their vaginal health and well-being.

Conclusion

As we come to the conclusion of this book, it's time to raise our glasses in celebration of the remarkable journey we've embarked upon—the journey towards happy, healthy "down there." So here's to you, dear reader, and to the incredible resilience and strength you've shown in embracing your body and taking charge of your vaginal health.

Imagine standing in front of a mirror, gazing at your reflection with newfound appreciation and love. Gone are the days of self-doubt and insecurity, replaced by a sense of empowerment and confidence in the skin you're in. You've learned to listen to your body's whispers, to honor its needs and desires, and to advocate fiercely for your own well-being. Today, you stand tall as the captain of your own vaginal ship, navigating the waves of life with grace and determination.

But let's not forget to acknowledge the challenges you've faced along the way—the moments of doubt, the setbacks, the times when it felt like the journey was too daunting to bear. Yet, through it all, you persevered. You sought knowledge, sought support, and most importantly, you never gave up on yourself. And for that, you deserve to be celebrated.

So here's to the countless Kegels you've done, strengthening your pelvic floor and safeguarding your vaginal health for years to come. Here's to the moments of mindfulness and meditation, where you found solace amidst the chaos of daily life and nurtured your mental and emotional well-being. Here's to embracing your body in all its imperfections, recognizing that true beauty lies in authenticity and self-acceptance.

However, our journey doesn't end here. In fact, it's only just beginning. As you step forward into the world armed with newfound knowledge and confidence, remember that you are never alone. You have a community of like-minded individuals standing beside you, ready to offer support, guidance, and encouragement every step of the way. Together, we can shatter the stigma surrounding vaginal health, rewrite the narrative, and create a world where every person's body is celebrated and respected.

As you reflect on the insights and knowledge gained from this book, I encourage you to take a moment to celebrate your journey towards vaginal wellness. Celebrate the small victories—the moments of self-discovery, the milestones achieved, the barriers overcome. Celebrate the courage it took to confront societal taboos and engage in open conversations about vaginal health. Most importantly, celebrate yourself—the incredible, resilient, and beautiful individual that you are.

Let this celebration not be the end of your journey, but rather the beginning of a new chapter. Let it serve as a reminder of your inherent worth and the power you possess to shape your own destiny. Let it inspire you to continue advocating for your own health and well-being, and to stand up against any forces that seek to diminish your worth or undermine your autonomy.

So here's to you, and to the journey that lies ahead. May it be filled with joy, fulfillment, and endless possibilities. May you always remember that your vagina, your body, and your life are yours to cherish, protect, and celebrate. Cheers to a happy, healthy "down there!"

www.ingramcontent.com/pod-product-compliance
Lightning Source LLC
Chambersburg PA
CBHW070926270326
41927CB00011B/2737